Healing While Writing

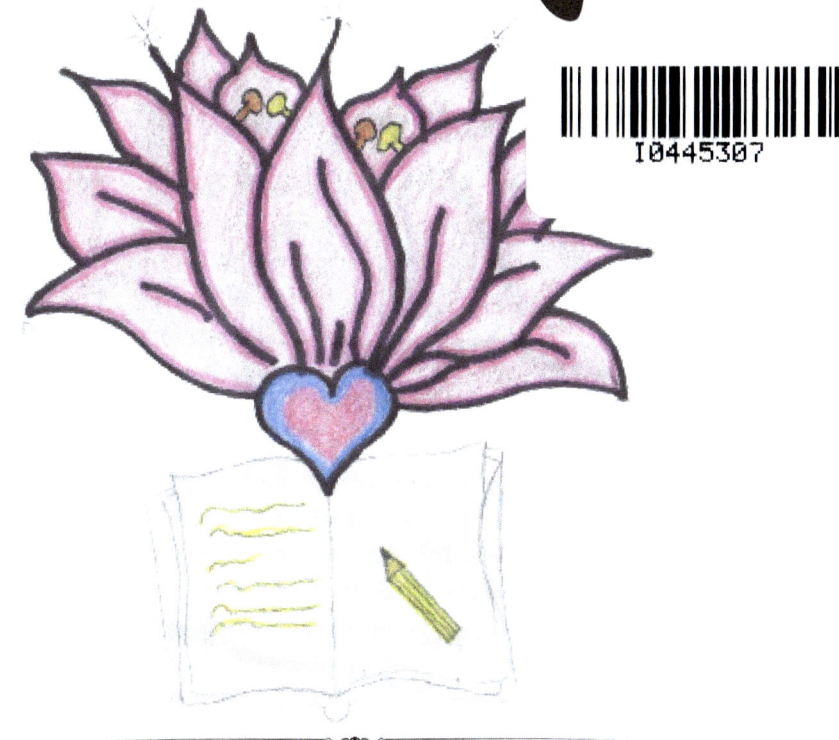

Grief Journal With Prompts
and Reflections
COVER BY: EDGARDO VELASQUEZ

CAROLINA AYALA-VELASQUEZ

Ordering Information:
Contact author at teamvelasquez@hotmail.com or order online
Instagram: Healing_while_hurting

Healing While Writing/Journal prompts and reflections / Carolina Ayala-Velasquez. —1st ed.

ISBN 979-8-9855006-3-9

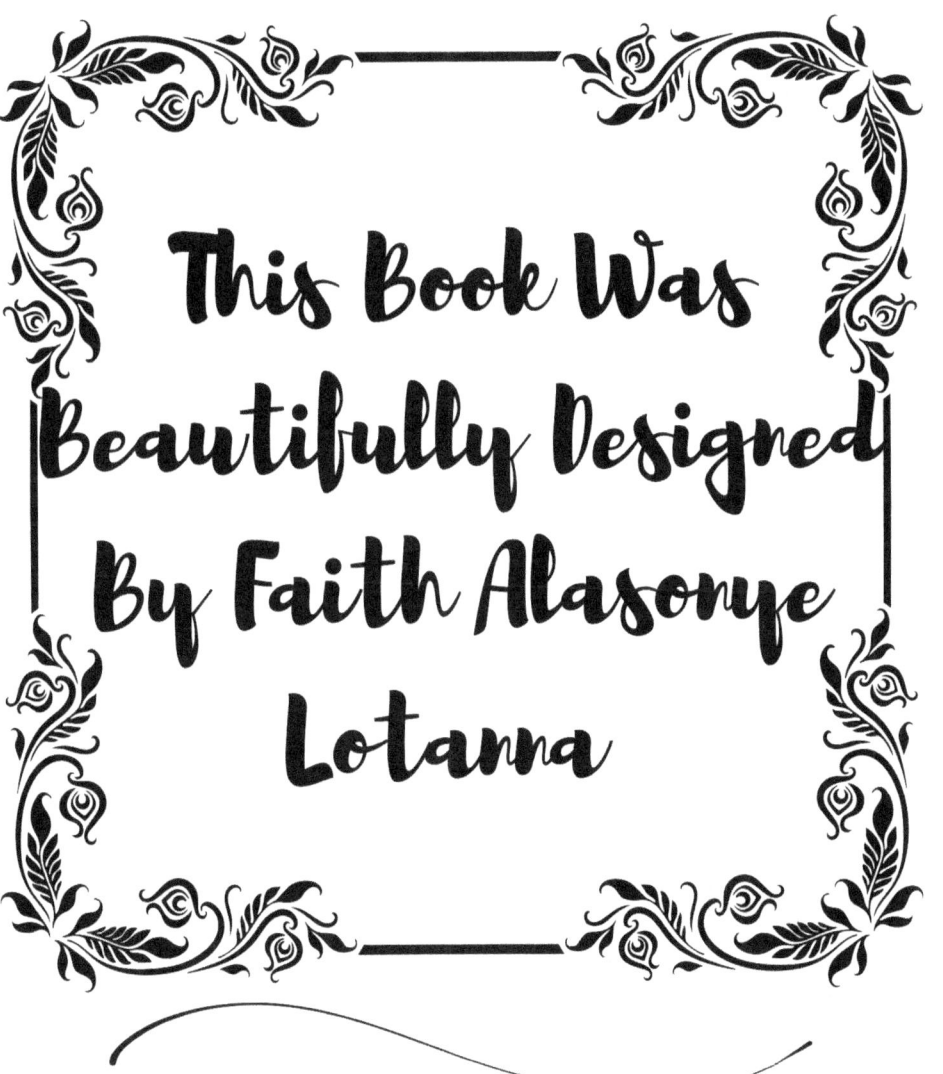

This Book Was Beautifully Designed By Faith Alasonye Lotanna

EMAIL: FALASONYELOTANNA@GMAIL.COM

PHONE CONTACT: +2348104323635

TABLE OF CONTENTS

Dedicated to my loved ones who have transitioned and my family that supports me on this journey.

The idea of this book was felt in my heart as a way to "accompany" my first ever self-published book "Healing While Hurting."
I was reminded I wanted to create a journal way back then within that book but decided it needed to be "separate." And now two years later, life brought me back to that original dream- with new transitions and visions.

I realize through that whole first book, the healing wasn't just from the hurt, it was through the writing.
Writing is one way I cope, heal and express myself.

While this book can "accompany" the first, it can also be just as powerful "on its own."
I hope this book helps you keep memories alive, love alive, hope alive, and healing happening.

I think there is something very powerful about showing up as you are; about being unpolished, unrehearsed and real. No one can tell your story like you can. We all have stories to tell. I think honesty creates opportunity for release and healing; and it also creates the space to make genuine connections. I thank you for being a part of making my dream a reality by supporting me on this author journey.

I am not just living a child-hood dream or life-long dream. I am living many dream come trues every time I get to create a book. I release with it's imperfections because I want you and everyone to know- you can create a book and live your dream without being "perfect", as long as it is good enough for you.

I am a life-long learner. I will continue to learn and grow and teach. I will continue to share my whole self, in hopes to inspire others to do the same
—May 18, 2022

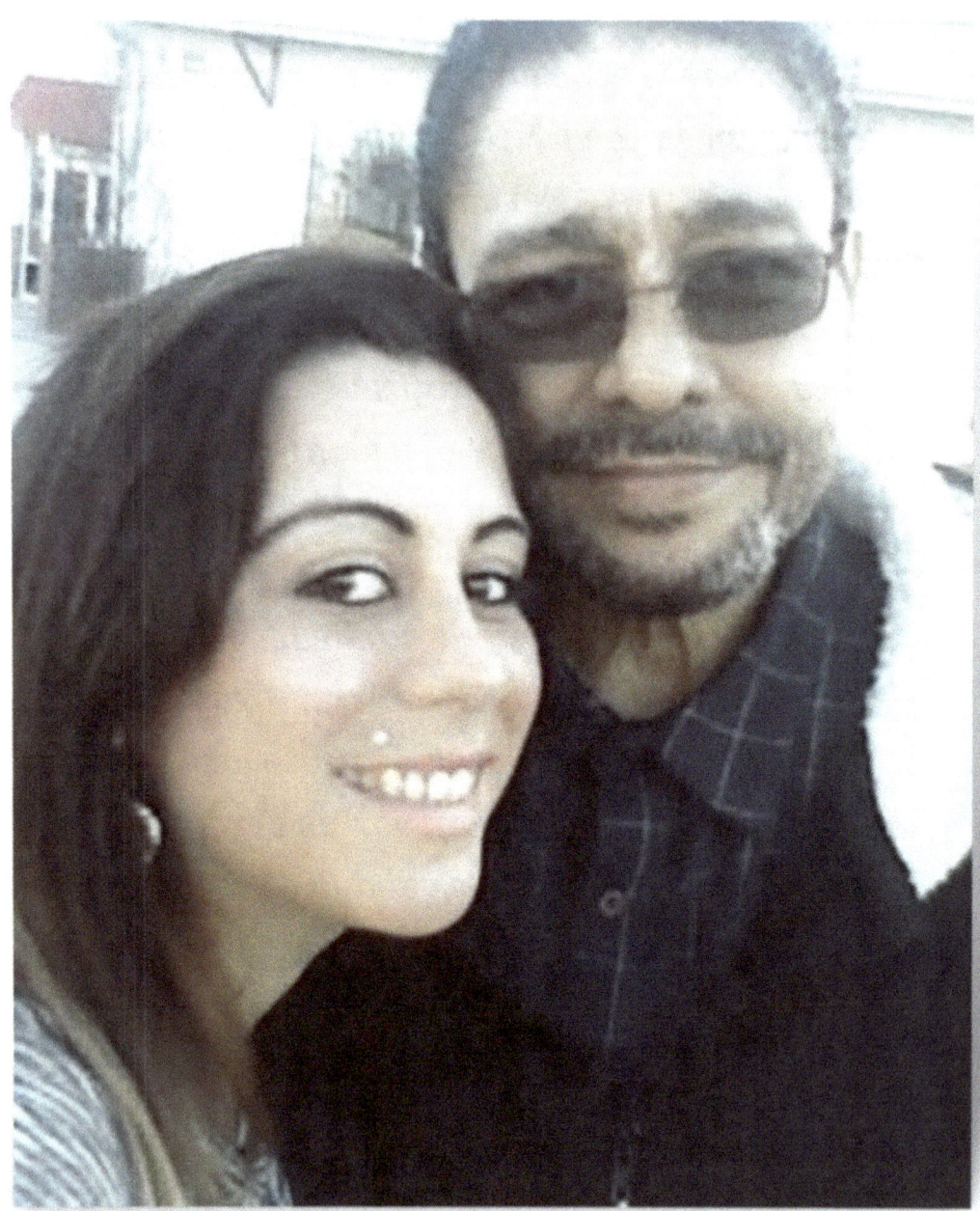

Juan Ramon Ayala

7/2/61-1/21/14

My dad. You leaving this earth in this way, was not the first time I have felt grief. But it was the first time the grief has stayed so long, hit me as hard and changed my whole world in so many layers because you aren't just my dad. You are the only grandfather my kids know. You are a father-in-law, brother, son, friend, uncle, cousin and so much more.

One lesson you taught me that I will always remember and teach others is "always wear your seatbelt, even if you are just going across the street." You said that to me once and it stuck. Sometimes I get sad knowing my future won't include you in the physical way it once did. Sometimes it hurts because I knew what life with you here did look like and it's easy to dream of what could've been.

The memories bring smiles and tears. Thank you for continuing to inspire and guide me. I love you. Always and forever, forever and always.

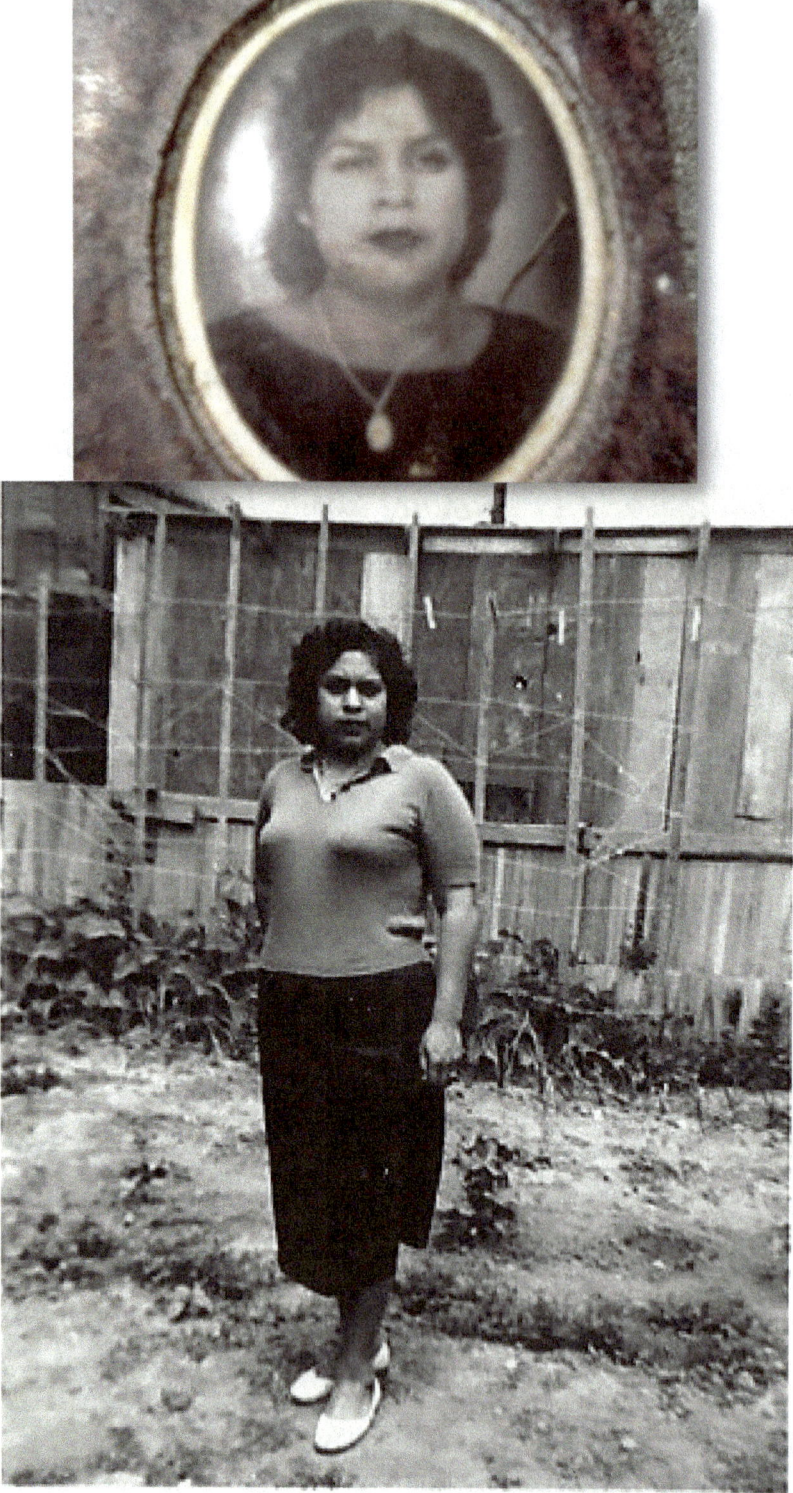

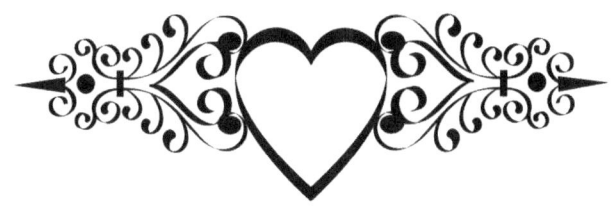

Lupe Rosalie Padilla is the name I have been told is yours. My father's mother. My grandmother who I am not sure I ever even knew.

I believe you passed when my dad was a child. In a car accident, I think. I don't know much about you at all. I am sorry I never asked questions, especially from my dad.

I wish I got to know you through him. I know he missed you. I know he loved you very much. I believe you are together now and I feel like he really needed you and now has you.

I am sorry I don't know you. But even in my not knowing, I pray for you and try to connect. I love you. Thank you for my father.

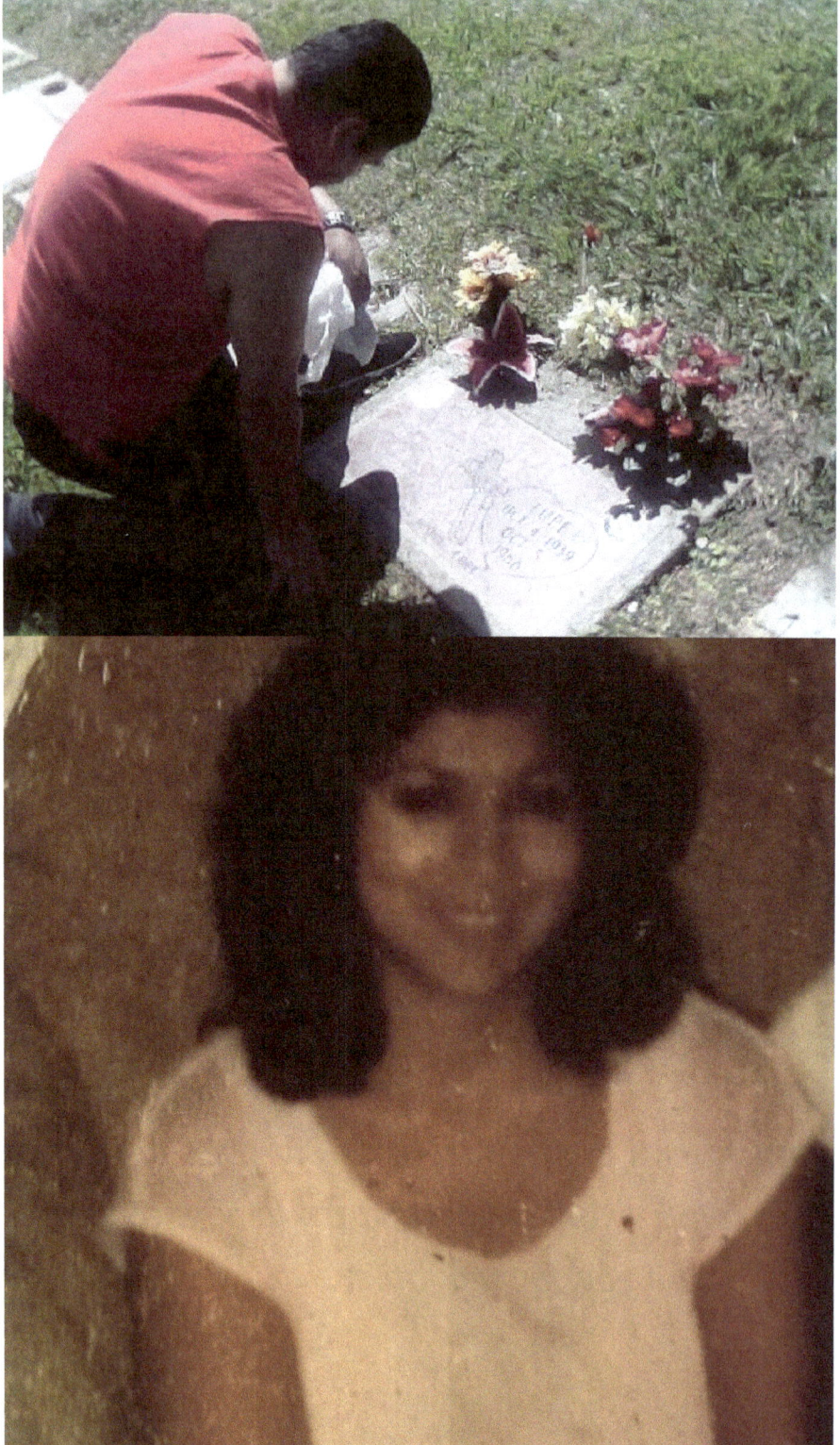

My aunty Pauline. I have maybe two pictures of us together and you were doing my hair as a baby.

Unfortunately, I do not have memories but I love when family share stories about you.

My dad always dedicated the sky to you on your birthday- the 4th of July, one of his favorite holidays. You meant so much to him and somehow that put you in my heart as if I knew you.

A younger me did. I Love you. Now you both can celebrate in the sky together.

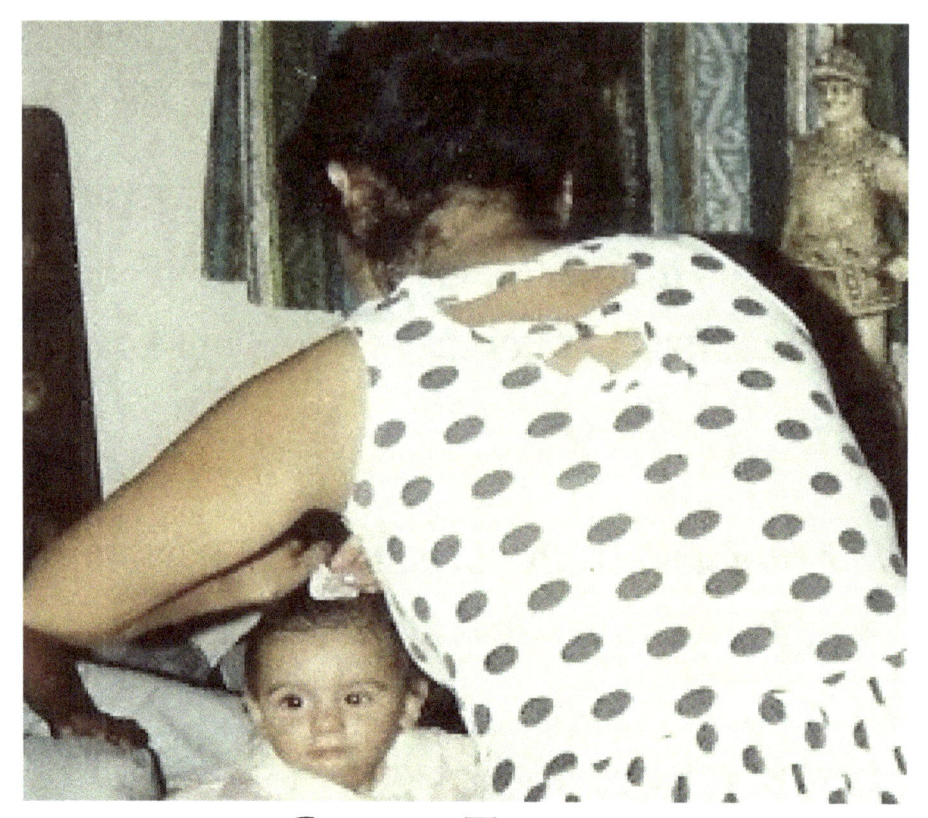

JUAN AYALA
July 4, 2011

Happy Birthday-To Pauline, Padilla-Galarza
(My sister who I LOVE And Miss SO MUCH)
R.I.P. LOVE YOU ALWAYS AND FOREVER...

The 4th of JULY just isn't the same without you...

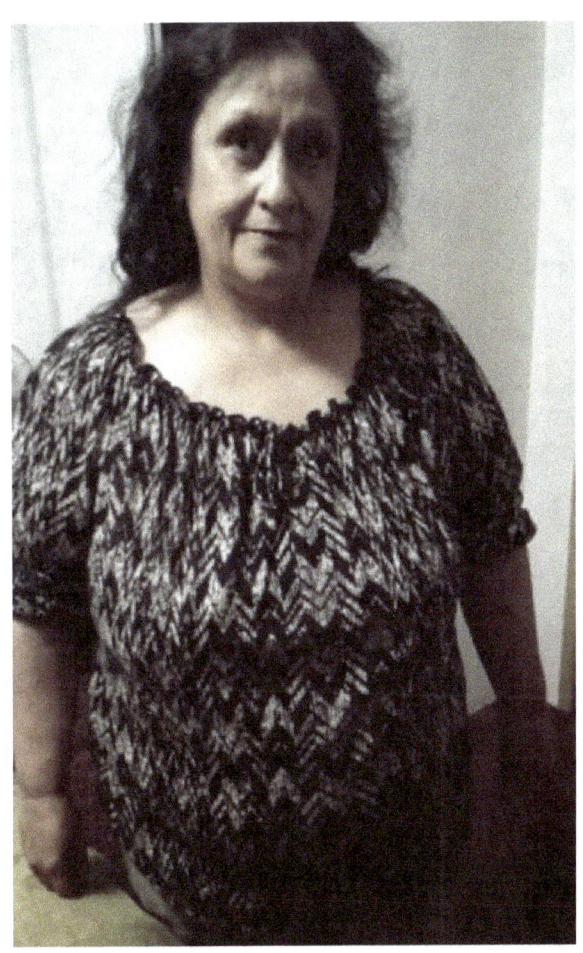

JENNIE LOUISE ORTIZ

JULY 31, 1959 – NOVEMBER 6, 2021

My dad's sister, my aunt.
11/14/21
Looking at pictures, I know this is my family
Looking at pictures, wondering.
Who is who, who is what to me
I see my dad in faces but yet so much is missing.
My condolences, my Aunty has joined my dad.
I wish I was closer; I really wish to build relationships.

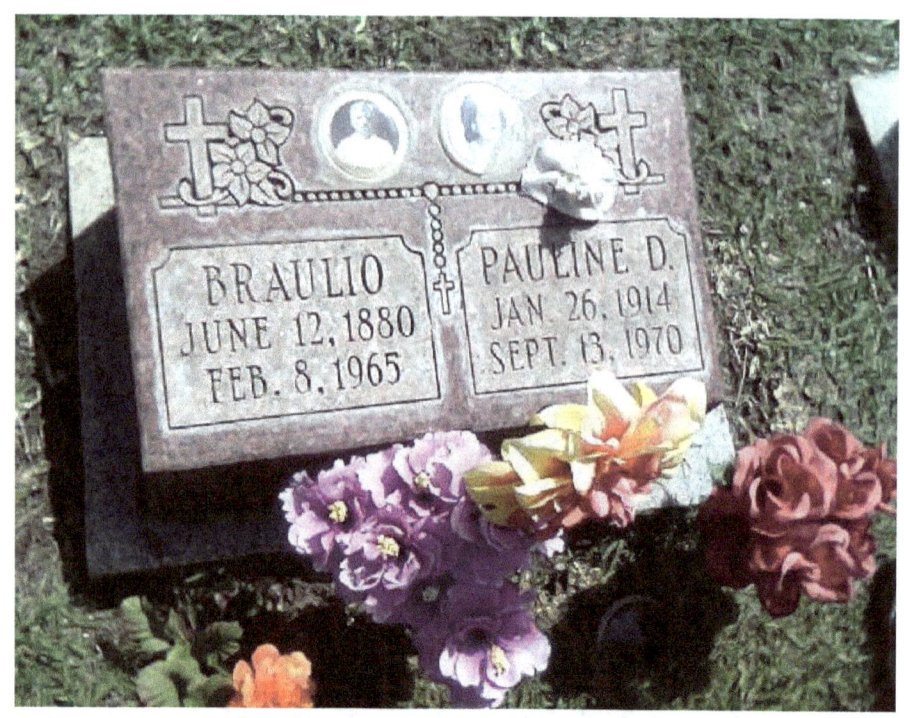

I am told you two are the parents of my grandpa Robert (who was really my dad's uncle/godfather which I didn't learn until I was much older.)

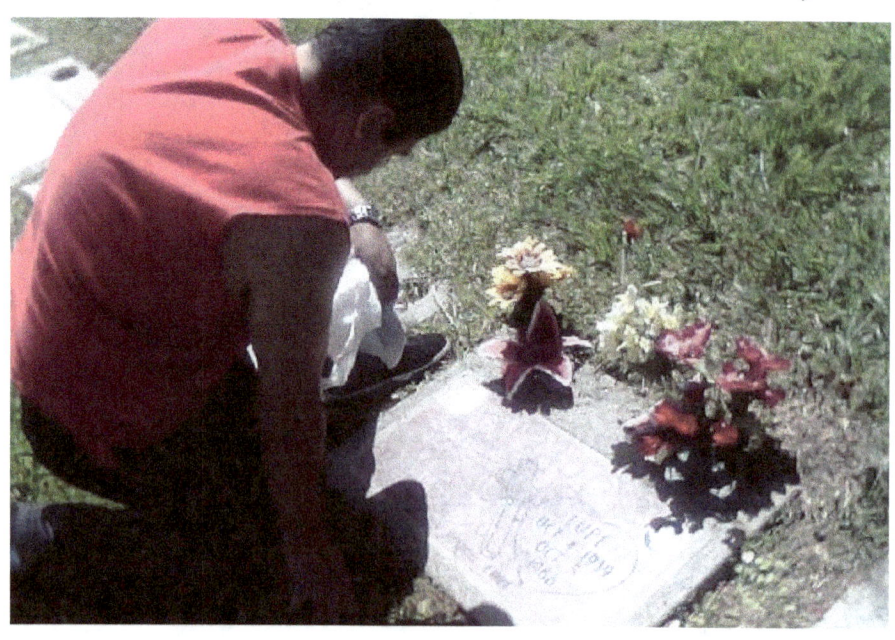

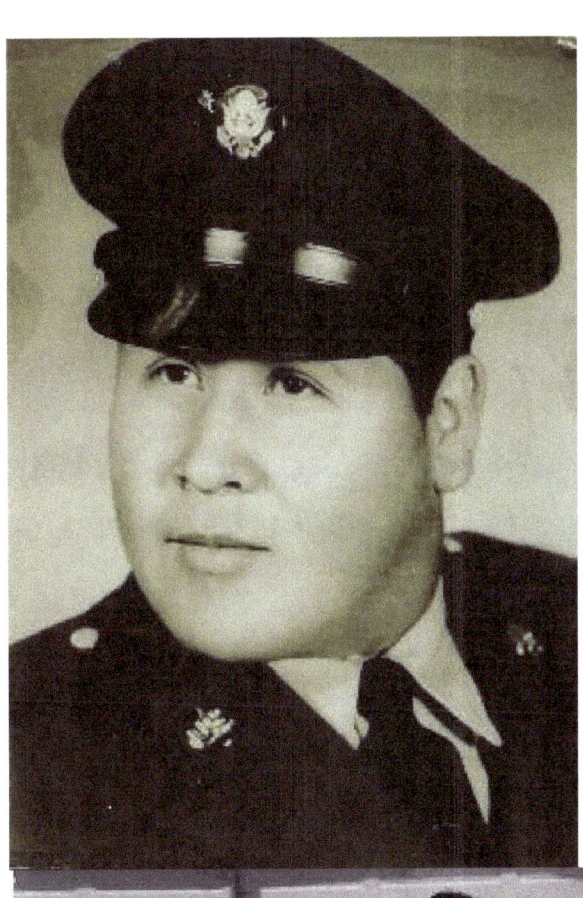

ROBERT DELGADO PADILLA,

MY GRANDFATHER

2/18/1941-9/27/2004

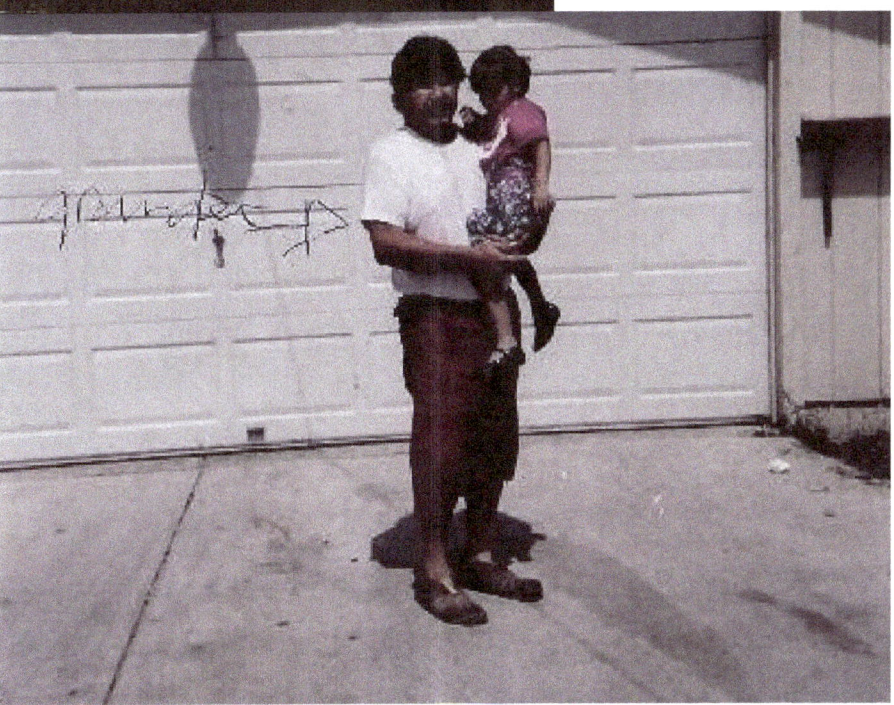

It isn't out of the ordinary that we would speak memories of my grandpa Robert when with my grandma and family.
But today my daughter asked how he died...
And I haven't felt that pain in a while.

I realized I had blocked some things away from my memory, but they aren't gone- they just went away for a long time.
Like him losing pieces of his body due to diabetes. Or even his eyesight.
So many triggered memories.
I never forgot about being at dialysis with him. Memories of making patients' drawings, and talking with them.
Memories of not knowing them as patients, just people.
Questions of the machines. Why is blood coming out, where is it going and why. And not knowing at that time that anything was really wrong.

I love hearing my grandma speak of him. The man he was. His humor. His heart.
I love seeing her face light up and hearing her laugh as she reminisces.

I'll always remember our trips to the doughnut shop on his bike and memories with my cousins about jalapeños, uncooked eggs, nightlights, and pull-ups.

Or how my cousin kept a picture of her mom on her mirror.

Or swimming with my uncle Larry.

Or the tire swing in the yard.

My grandma made her famous salsa that my daughter now loves. My daughter and I added extra serrano's even though she said it was spicy already.

She couldn't believe it.

I said "well, I grew up on jalapenos. I learned it here" 😎 ❤️

It feels so good to have made the time to be here tonight.

Even with the sad moments.

Thankful. For family, memories, love, support, food and time together.

9/27/14
GRANDPA ROBERT

10 years ago, I lost someone who meant the world to me, my grandpa Robert. I found out with a phone call while I was in school and I just remember breaking down right then and there on the phone falling to my knees, tears falling uncontrollably. I was 15. I didn't get to say goodbye. I felt like I wasn't important enough to get a call to go say goodbye, I felt hurt, I felt like all I wanted was to tell him how much I love him.

After losing my dad this year and being there until the last breath, being able to say goodbye was the hardest thing I ever had to do but I made sure to call as many people as I could because he wanted and deserved to be surrounded by love and I didn't want anyone to feel that feeling I held of not being able to say goodbye-or not being thought of to be given the chance. I was thankful I was able to go with family on the boat to spread your ashes.it was a special, very sad moment.

I never questioned the title grandpa.
As I got older, I was told he wasn't really my grandpa-he's my dad's uncle and as I was told this I remember saying no-you are my grandpa and you will be forever.
I was a baby when I was told he was my grandpa and even as I'm older-that is who you will forever be to me and I thank my dad for making you that in my life.

I remember living with you when I was little, going to preschool from your house, riding on the back of your bike going to the doughnut shop every morning, playing on the tire swing in the backyard, walking on your back to crack your back, watching all of the Disney movies while you sat in your chair.

I use to spend early mornings going with you to dialysis and walking around making cards for all of the people there and I would hear you just brag about how special I was and how much you loved me. I remember your smile, your voice, and your hugs.

You always made sure to come to my birthday parties after I moved back with my mom. You would take me school shopping for whatever I needed and wanted. As I got older and you got sick I was told you would forget who I was but even after time apart and as you got sicker my last memory-you remembered me after they said you wouldn't. I cooked eggs for you like you use to for me, with your crushed ice and water.

Not a single day goes by that I don't miss you. Every visit to the house to see grandma is hard with you not there and I always have flashbacks to the way the house used to be.

Sitting on the washer and dryer helping grandma fold laundry, doing handstands in the living room where the big mirror use to be on the wall.

You will forever be such a huge part of my heart. I love you. Thank you for so many of my best memories as a child. I cherish so much dearly.

2/18/20

Anyone missing someone today?

I am
Thought of you at 1am and throughout the day.
I should have called to check on grandma but I couldn't bring myself to do it.
I got sad thinking about you and missing you.
I tried to smile at the good memories.
You gave me so much and I don't think you'll ever know just how much you gave and mean to me.
Thank you for being there for my dad, for taking me in when my parents needed help. For being my grandpa - I would have grown up without one but instead GOD gave me you.

I know to many, the facts matter (that you were my dad's uncle/godfather and not my biological grandfather) but to me those facts will never be what matters. To my heart and my whole growing up- you are and always will be my grandpa Robert. The only one I had, such a blessed grandpa at that. I feel even more fortunate that the role and title was a chosen one because you didn't have to do that.

From the morning bike rides to the doughnut shop, to you getting upset making us eggs we asked for but didn't like and asking me to jump on your back. You guys always would buy me what I didn't have and what I needed. I would love being able to eat jalapenos with you because my only access was at your house- I never knew I could get them anywhere else lol.

I loved watching tv with you. So many memories that mean everything. Like old cowboy shows and golden girls with grandma.
Thank you for loving me.
I am so thankful to have you, grandma, my cousins growing up and still.
You all have truly made my life so much more special and meaningful.

Happy heavenly birthday to my grandpa Robert. Thankful for so much. 1 person can give you so many reasons to be grateful.

2/18/11

Pictures are all I have left visually, memories stay in my brain and heart. you never leave my mind, the bracelet in your remembrances never left my wrist, a shirt in your memory for my graduation, pictures, and a poem on my wedding day.

Pictures/momentums from your funeral, stories grandma tells me. I COULD NEVER FORGET YOU. I would never want to, the only grandpa I've ever known. I LOVE YOU MORE THAN WORDS CAN SAY. Happy bday grandpa Robert .r.i.p

9/28/17

I woke up this morning from a crazy dream, I wouldn't say it was a good one- I was angry with a lot of people, and although for good reason, it wasn't a good dream.....

However in this dream, in a crowd of people was this man, this young man, and I just knew that I knew him...it was my grandpa but at this time he must not have been my grandpa, it was like his eyes knew who I was but nothing else about him knew me, we just stared for a moment and then the dream continued...but I know it was him.....
he hasn't been in my dreams for a very long time, what a nice surprise

9/27/17

In 2004 I lost a man who meant the world to me. It hit me like a ton of bricks. This loss was my greatest loss at that time and for a long time in my life. My dad reminded me so much of my grandpa Robert. I still wear my bracelet, from my grandmother that she made after he passed. It never comes off, in memory of him.

Some of my greatest early childhood memories were when I was with him and my grandma. I remember getting that call more than I do of actually going on the boat to spread his ashes. I remember it being so hard to go around after he passed. He spoiled me with movies and shopping and a good life anytime I was with them. I am forever thankful for the man he was and I am forever grateful for all he did for me.

To this day those memories help mold me. I remember thinking I'll never forget my best friend's birthday with such a devastating situation to happen. My grandpa was a great man. I still have money he collected during the war and anytime I'm with my grandma and family we talk of the stories and memories and it always feels so good.

I miss the lemon tree and the forever supply of jalapeños. He was the man who would put soap in your mouth if you cursed, the man who made the 4th of July unforgettable, and the man who loved his family to the fullest. The way my grandparents fought for me, loved me, took care of me, and listened is something will forever appreciate. I miss you, grandpa.

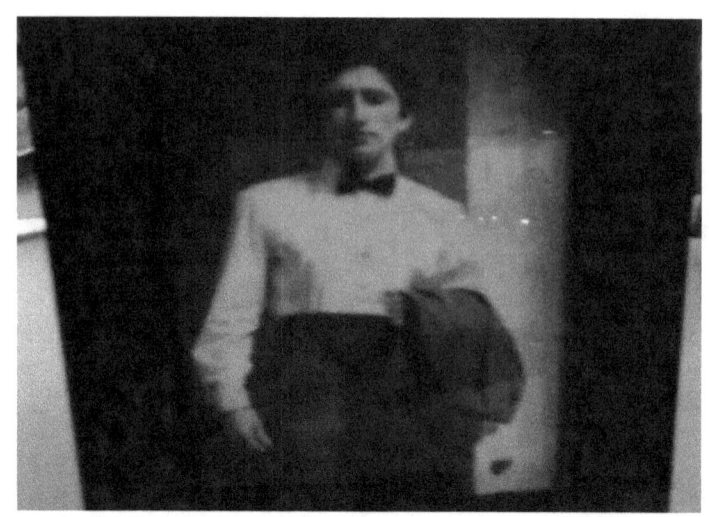

I will always know you as my uncle Larry. And the one memory I have that has forever stayed was when we went swimming at a pool one day. You, your girlfriend and both of my cousins. I was maybe 6 or younger. I remember being scared to go on the floating bed and my cousins really wanted me to.

I

remember falling off and not being able to swim. I remember being told you jumped in to save me, that I almost drowned.

I have stories of you, others told. But none I know or remember for myself.

Thank you. For saving me, for taking me to have fun and I am sorry you had to go before your parents.

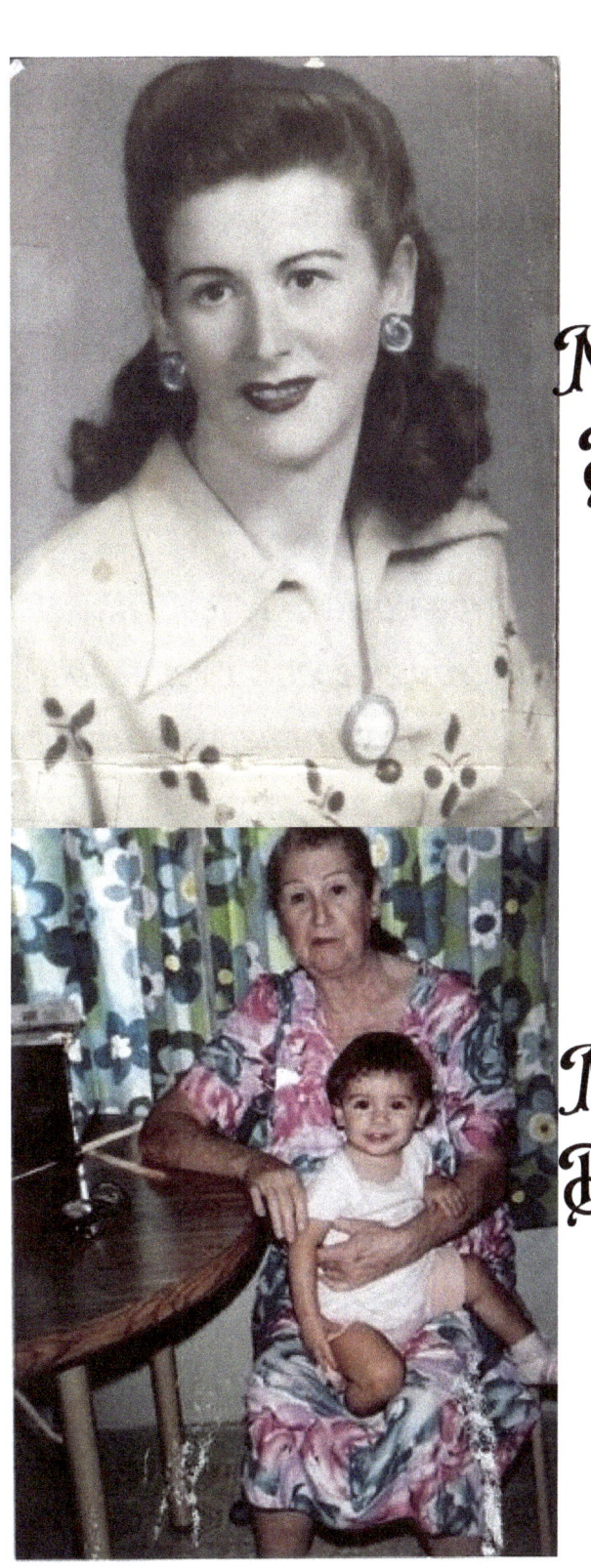

MADELEINE DONOHUE

MADELEINE DONOHUE

JULY 28, 1923-
DECEMBER 11, 1993

My mom's mom, my grandmother.
Your name is my middle name. My oldest brother has the most memories with and of you. I have very few pictures and the memories are not there.

I wish I had more memories. I feel like I remember you had a strong accent. I remember you cooking. I feel like I even remember living with you at some point. I am not sure how much I remember or if I made it up from pictures but I feel connected to you. As I have gotten older, I feel like I started losing you, pieces that I once knew and could feel- smell even. They just disappeared. And now, I am trying to get back to all I lost.

A native of France. Longtime resident oA longtimed. You had a brother named Pierre. A mother of 7. You were cremated and your ashes live at my aunt's home.

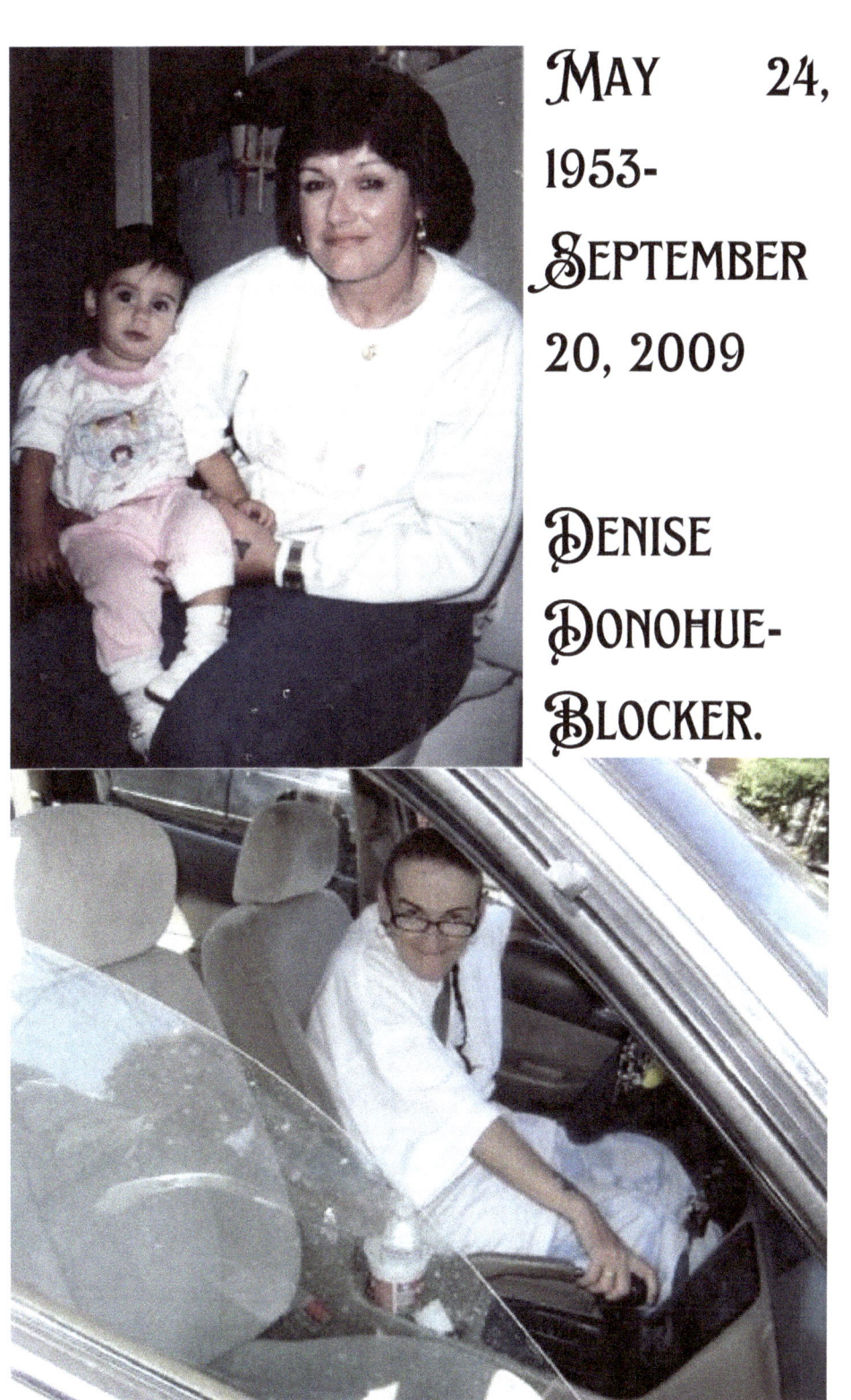

MAY 24, 1953- SEPTEMBER 20, 2009

DENISE DONOHUE-BLOCKER.

My mom's sister. My aunt.

Why don't we have more pictures together? As I got older. We lived together at several times. You and my mom were so close forever, all of life when you were here. You were always here or we would always be visiting you.

I use to love when you would do my hair. Any style but I loved braids.

It was so hard watching you get sick, watching you slip away.

I remember that call.... I remember you not wanting to stay here earthside anymore.... because of what your body was going through.

I remember my mom losing her best friend. That was one of the hardest things to see, my moms' pain. You were always a protector, willing to fight any fight for yourself or those you love.

The two pictures chosen, I feel like you were very different versions of yourself and yet your heart never changed and neither did your spunk.

I love the grandmother you were, more like mom. You always loved generously and with all of you.

Homegoing Celebration

for

Curtis Wayne Blocker, Jr.

Sunrise: June 20, 1970   Sunset: January 26, 2002

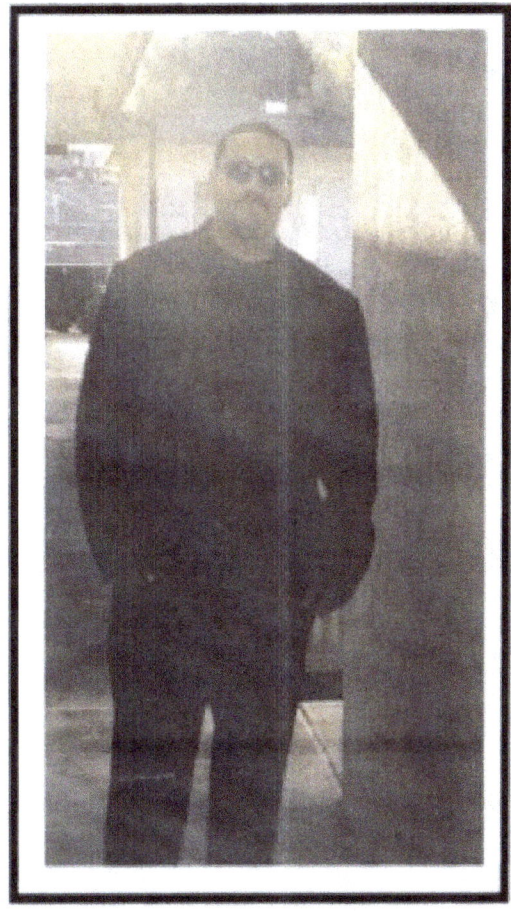

Hudson Fouche's Funeral Home
3665 Telegraph Avenue
Oakland, California 94609
Tuesday February 5, 2002
Officiating
Rev. Henry Shepard

My cousin Wayne. My aunt Denise's son.

We have no pictures together, even though I remember taking pictures of you with my camera back then. I remember when you would visit and the laughs my mom would have. I remember your funeral and how "huge" it was. Like a celebrity. I remember how hurt my aunt, my uncle and cousins were when you left this earth. How hurt they still are.

I see so much of you in your children, my cousins.

You live on through all who miss and love you and continue to share about you.

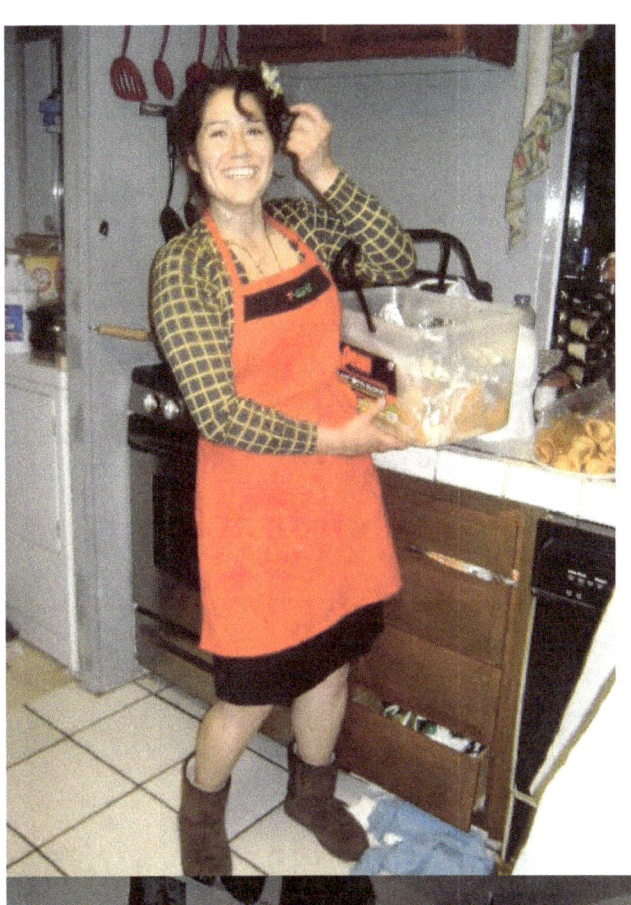

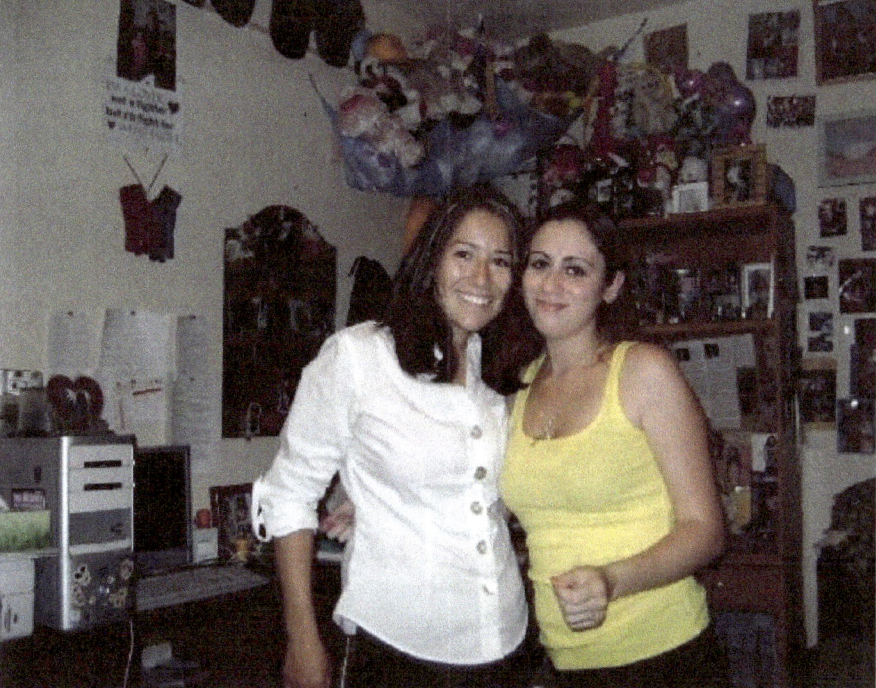

11/20/13

They say today makes 2 years since you been gone...i found out on the 21st two years ago...i cant believe how much time has passed with you gone. Most days I dont feel like you are gone. Every day I know it, there's still many days tears fall and candles get lit and I talk to the sky for you.

So thankful for memories, goodtimes, pictures and being spiritual. I love you Jossie. You will never be forgotten. You will forever live on. I know you lay to rest in Mexico but you are very much stil here around me daily.

Rest in paradise sis, keep watching over us.

1/8/10

Everything takes time but time flies. Don't wait until later, do what you want and need to, now. Later may never come. Later may come and you don't want to be stuck in the same place you are now. Time passes by so fast, so live for today, live for tomorrow and be ok with your past cause life is too short.

I'm not sure when I'll believe it, when it will hit me hardest-that you're not here anymore. I'm so off and on with the breaking down. Sometimes I'm a mess and other minutes I don't even believe it. I'm glad we have so many memories. I am glad so many have so many memories with you.

My love and prayers to your family.

1.1.05

It's too easy to fall into depression when you have a situation in life that hurts you. It makes it too easy to think of all the bad. I have to remember some things we can't control and its ok to hurt but don't fall apart and have more to add to the list of depression.

Reminding myself to stay positive and always look toward the good. It was very hard to be in class, I heard nothing the teacher even said. My mind is on Jossie, on life, on death, too many thoughts. Too many questions, too many unknowns, waiting on answers and questioning if I can even believe any of it. It hits me off and on, that it's real.

I still feel like it can't be...just can't be

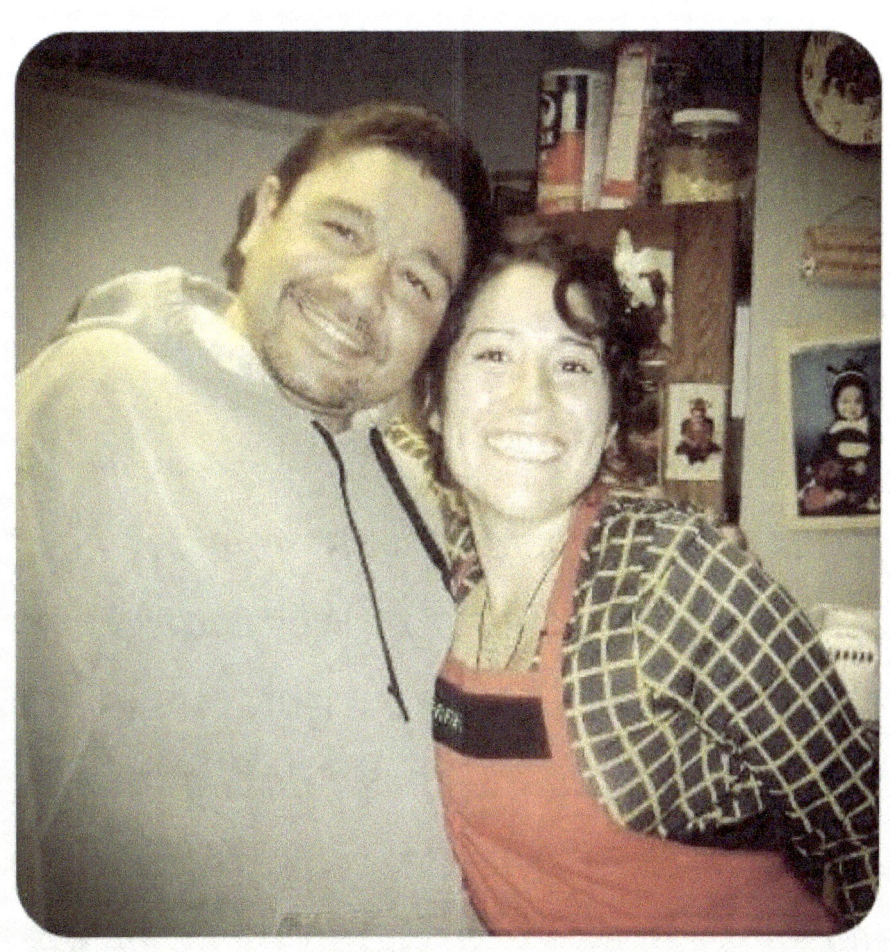

1.1.2005

I had never dyed my hair before-with you we did it together.

you showed me how to put on cover up makeup and to cut my eyebrows. We went to kings boxing together. When you needed a place to stay, you moved in with me and we became family.

I remember teaching you how to make that day was funny. We shared my clothes/shoes/room. You got me to try tofu, you helped me sneak hubby into the house back in the day lol. We had so many good times, so many pictures, and so much fun.

So many memories. And I am stuck here, can't get it all of my mind and heart.

7/7/67 - 10/24/22

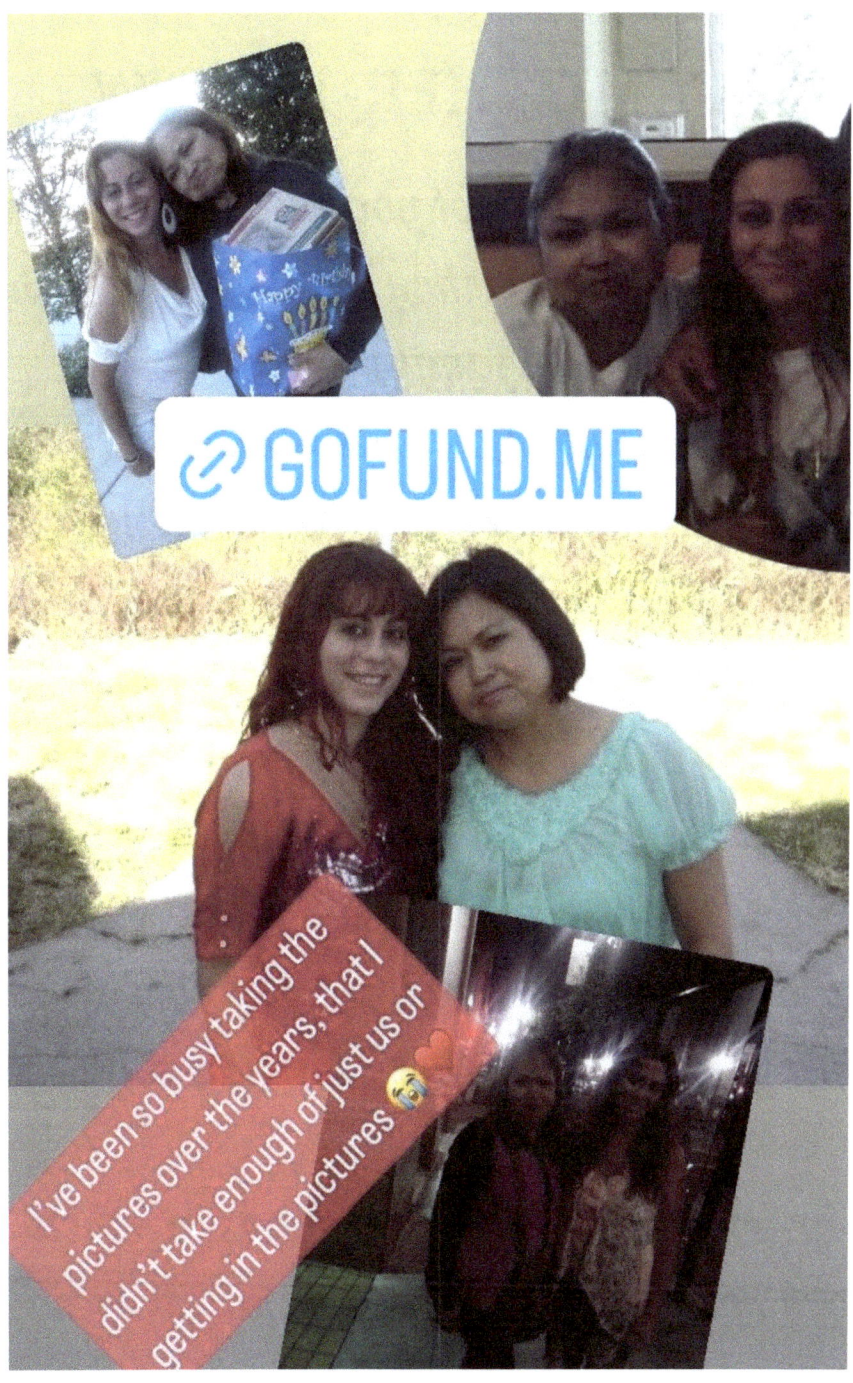

GOFUND.ME

I've been so busy taking the pictures over the years, that I didn't take enough of just us or getting in the pictures 😭

Martha Alicia Mora Castorena

MY MOTHER-IN-LAW

Some who never met you but know of you through us, say they saw you as the matriarch of the family.

When someone you love has uncurable cancer, you know your time is limited- you just don't know what that will mean or look like. You are still never prepared.

Thank you for all you brought into my world and life with your humor, culture, guidance, faith, and love. Thank you for being the grandmother only you could be.

My mother-in-law, my sponsor when I was being baptized- I love and appreciate you.

Lena Ayala-Velasquez
October 17, 2022 ·
Shared with Your friends

I can't believe I'm seeing this and it's now real in this way.

To my friends and family , who I can now share with.

Yes, my birthday was this weekend.

I spent the day with my family as we took on the new journey of my amazing mother-in-law being transferred to a hospice facility.

If I haven't responded to birthday wishes, it's because that day and all weekend we have been processing so much.

My mother-in-law has been battling cancer for some years now. And she keeps surpassing what any doctors say is "her time"

She is strong, she is a fighter, she has faith.

She is also tired and we know this road is on its journey to the next transition.

Lena Ayala-Velasquez
3/3/16

Thank you to my mother in law. For doing my hair for our wedding, for doing the girls hair. Thank you for the beautiful flower pen favors. For watching Leo everyday while we work. For always having a hot meal ready, dishes clean and everything. You ask for nothing from us. You moved in back in June and we love having you around, not because of what you do for us. We love having you, your presence, your knowledge, your jokes, your love. The kids are speaking Spanish, my husband is so happy to have his mom everyday, I'm thankful to have such a awesome motherinlaw. Daily coffee, flowers here and there- all of that is nothing compared to what you mean to us. We love you so much. So happy to have you around. So grateful for all you do for us,help us with. Your support and love mean so much. All we want is to see you happy, to help and support when you need it, to give you a life you deserve because you deserve the best.

You are such a strong, beautiful person inside and out.

(May 9, 2021)To my mother-in-law, I love you. Excited to see you today. Without you, I have no husband and no children that I do, today. Happy mothers day. Thank you for your son. Thank you for the grandmother you are to our children. Thank you for being such a strong, loving, and powerful woman, mom, and mother-in-law. we love you

(4/6/16)My mother-in-law amazes me...she watches the kids all day while we work. Right now she can't work but really wants to. She doesn't expect or ask for anything from us. She goes to school and then comes home to still take care of the kids, bathing the baby. Not everyone is fortunate enough to have a woman like her around. She is so strong, selfless, happy, and amazing.

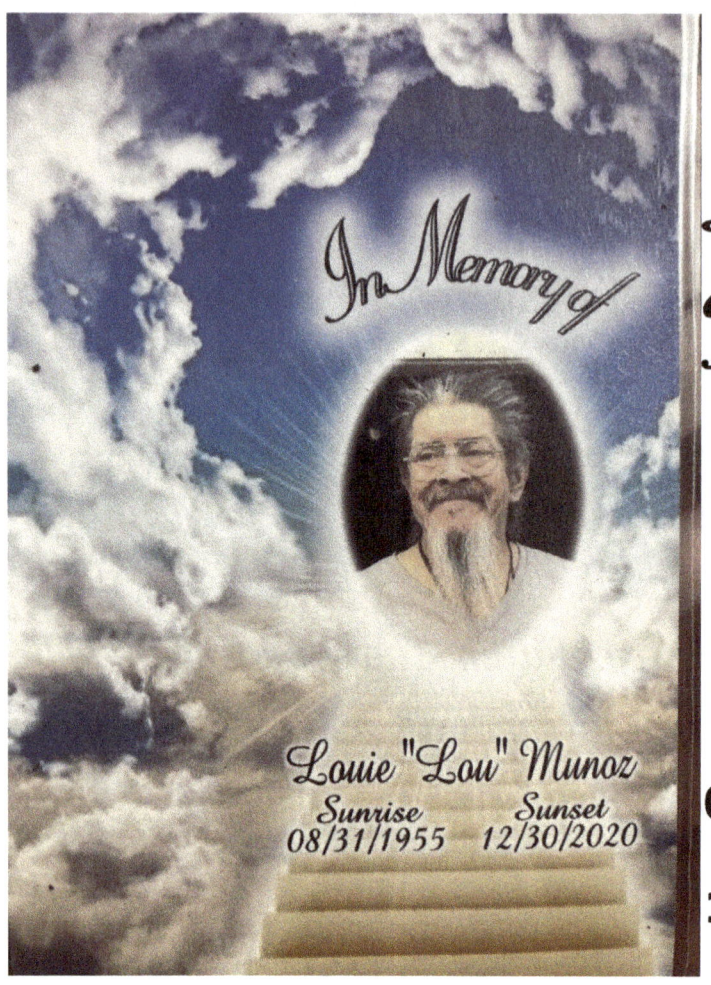

Louie "Lou" Munoz
Sunrise   Sunset
08/31/1955   12/30/2020

LOUIE MUNOZ

08/31/1955
-
12/30/2020

I have known Louie since I was a child, probably since I was born. The pain in my nini's voice when she told me he passed, is a sound I feel like I will never forget. Sending so much love to his children, grandchildren ,and my nini: Darlene.

What I will remember is his smile, his chill attitude ,and the way he loved his family. I can still hear his voice and am thankful for who he was in this lifetime.

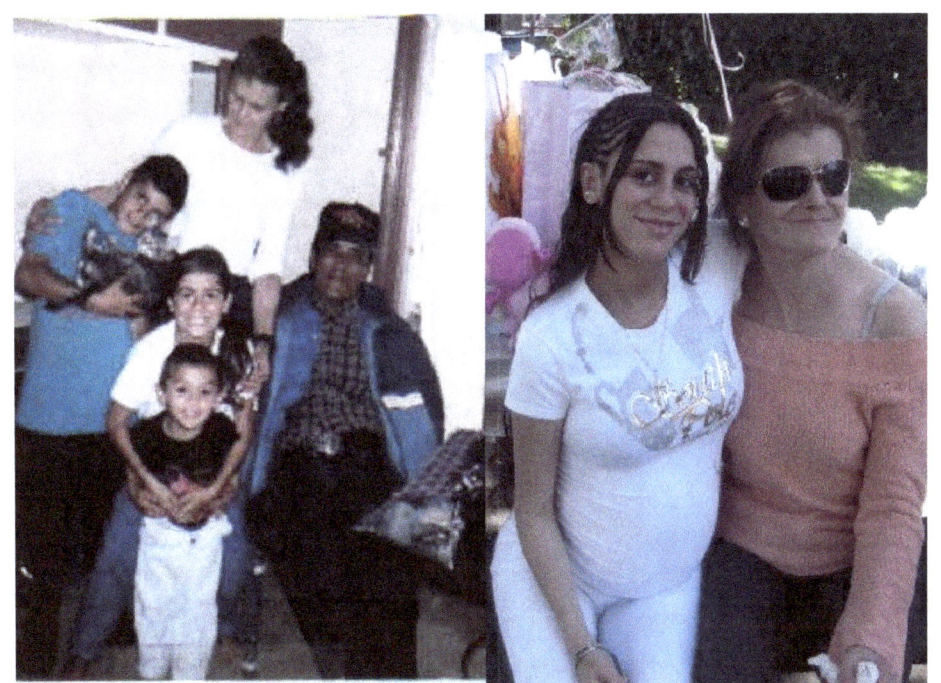

Gilbert and Earlene Fernandez. Gilbert passed away when I was a lot younger. I don't remember the date. And Earlene passed away December 22, 2022. I have known them since I was a very young child, I feel like they were always there.

We lived together for a long time and even when we didn't, we were always together for what feels like a big amount of my childhood. We are family, forever. Although I didn't see you much these past handful of years, my mom remained very close.

I am sure you and Gilbert are together again. I know your sons and family will miss you.

I know my mom will miss you.

We love you.

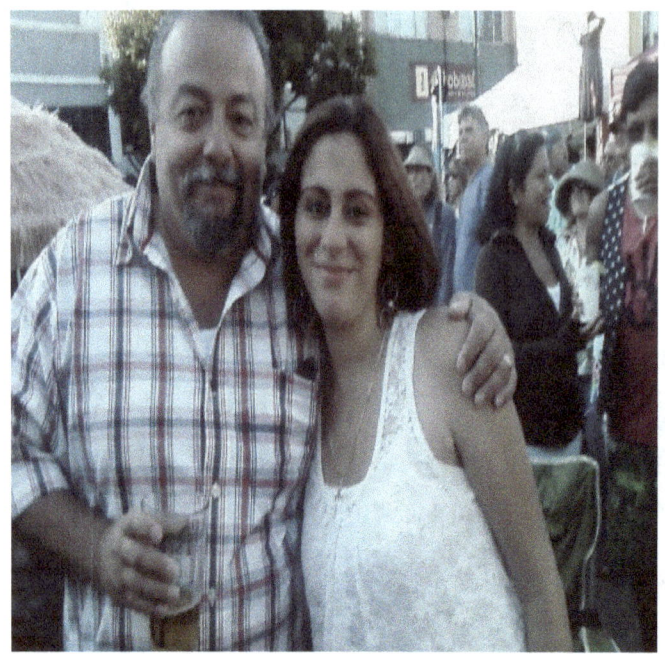

My uncle.
My aunt Louise's Husband.
My moms brother-in-law.

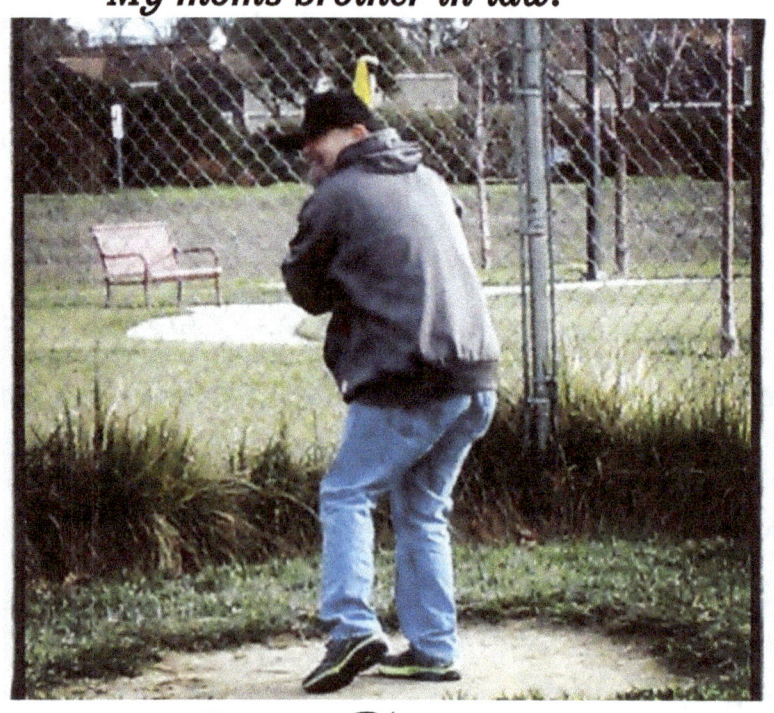

John Vasquez

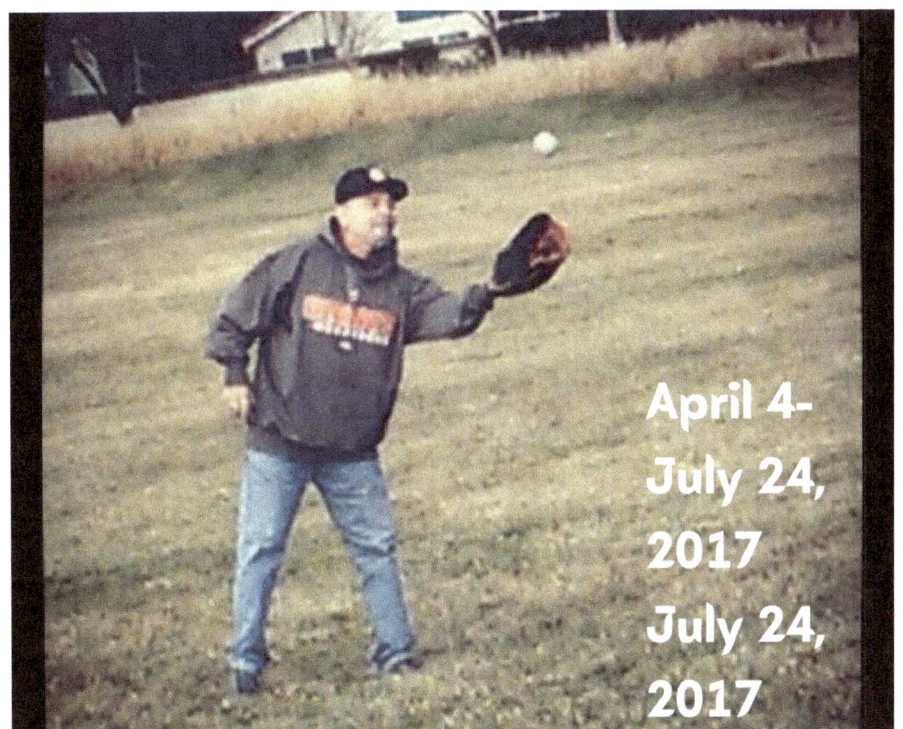

April 4-
July 24,
2017
July 24,
2017

The day was flying by really fast. 2 hours before work was going to be over I found out my uncle passed away. I was/am heartbroken. It made those 2 hours longer. I cried some tears without the kids noticing, they were busy on the beach. I held it together but I am so very hurt. He had cancer, he knew this time was coming but yet you never know when. Although we knew it was coming-you can never prepare for the heartache and surprise and pain. We were blessed to make memories with him over the years. He always had a smile, always jokes and stories to tell. He was always kind and such a gentleman. He greeted me with a hug and was always checking in on everyone.

He played baseball with my kids, golf with my husband. He is an outstanding role model of what a man should be. Such an amazing father and husband. Our last memories are from a few weeks ago, he was tired but still trying to make coffee for everyone and not relax. We spent time on the couch. He asked me about my dad, about his final days and how he looked/felt. He said he was feeling similar.

He

spoke about this with such calmness and I spoke without tears trying to be realistic and hopeful. I love you uncle John. I cant believe you are gone. Such a beautiful soul. You didn't deserve the pain and suffering and I am happy you no longer have to endure that. But I am so sad that the world lost someone so very valuable, loved and beautiful. You made and will continue to make the world a better place. You live on through every life you touched and believe me the amount of people you have impacted is enormous.

Today is the service for my uncle John. As much as we want to be there to say our last goodbye and support my cousins and aunt...I know they are surrounded by people, love, family, and support. The kids haven't been to a funeral since my dad passed away, and I feel it would be too much for them. On top of wanting to be local for my mother-in-law.

Today we celebrated my uncle's life and memory at the art and wine festival because this is an event he loved and attended often. This time, we sit with our last memories of him from weeks ago and the past. I am happy he was around to see the digital frame and give us so many great memories to cherish.

Uncle john we love you so much, we will miss you. To my cousins and aunt, I love you so much and can definitely relate to the loss of losing an amazing father. I know there is nothing I can do or say to make it better, we send our love and prayers. Your smile, kindness, love of golf and giants, love for family, your cooking, your hospitality, your heart- forever lives on.

we listened to Santana music with my uncle at the festival. My uncle would always come to the art and wine festival.

This is how we remember him and celebrate his life. He would be here with a drink, smiling, listening to music, then come sit on the stairs to talk and laugh before driving back home.

August 11, 2017

I had a dream about my uncle john last night. (It must have been because the kids were talking about wanting to visit aunty Louise.) the kids went running into their house wanting to tell uncle john something, knowing he passed but it not registering he wouldn't be there to talk to. We all fell to the floor crying, coping with the fact that he is no longer there to talk to.

That's all I remember of my dream but it is for certain that my uncle left a mark on me, my husband and our kids-he was like having a grandpa around when theirs passed. He is uncle john to us all.

He gave us so much care and love and memories to hold in our hearts. Although death is a part of "life" -it is hard to grasp when loved ones mean so much to us.

Forever in our hearts uncle John. and so much love for my aunty. hopefully, we will see you sometime soonish. We love you.

April 4, 2018.

Sending love to my aunt and cousins. I know it's not easy and it doesn't necessarily ever get easier. Thank you for all the memories uncle John, of golfing with my husband, baseball with us and the kids, buying lemonade from the kid's lemonade stand, and listening to music at the art and wine fair.

You always had a smile and hug for all of us.

You were always working, doing chores, cooking, cleaning, and always busy.

You are now in heaven, with my dad. You will forever be a great man, person, husband, father, uncle, friend.... everything. You were the best role model to all.

I love you. We miss you.

Thank you for being the strong, beautiful, thoughtful, respectful, and funny soul you are.

You live on.

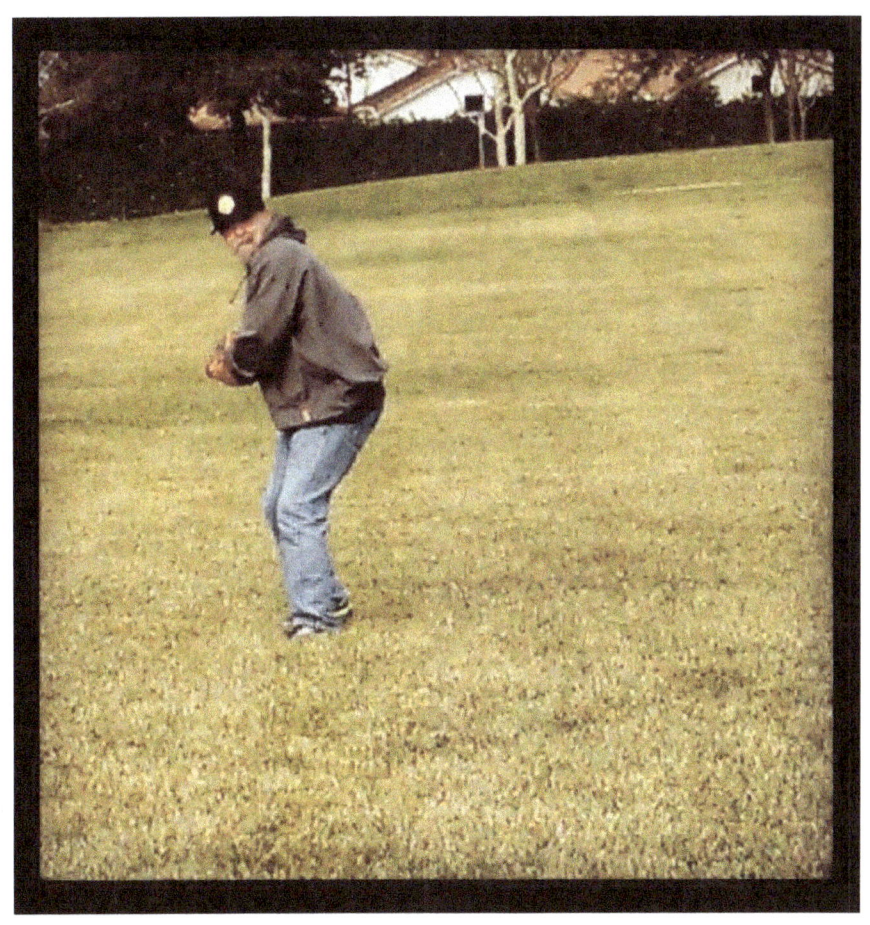

I miss his voice, positive energy, hugs, smile and the role model he was.

Missing my own dad, I'm constantly thinking of my cousins and aunt and wishing them well because I know how hard it is.
I know there's nothing no one can do or say. But I love you all and he lives on through everyone he's ever met.

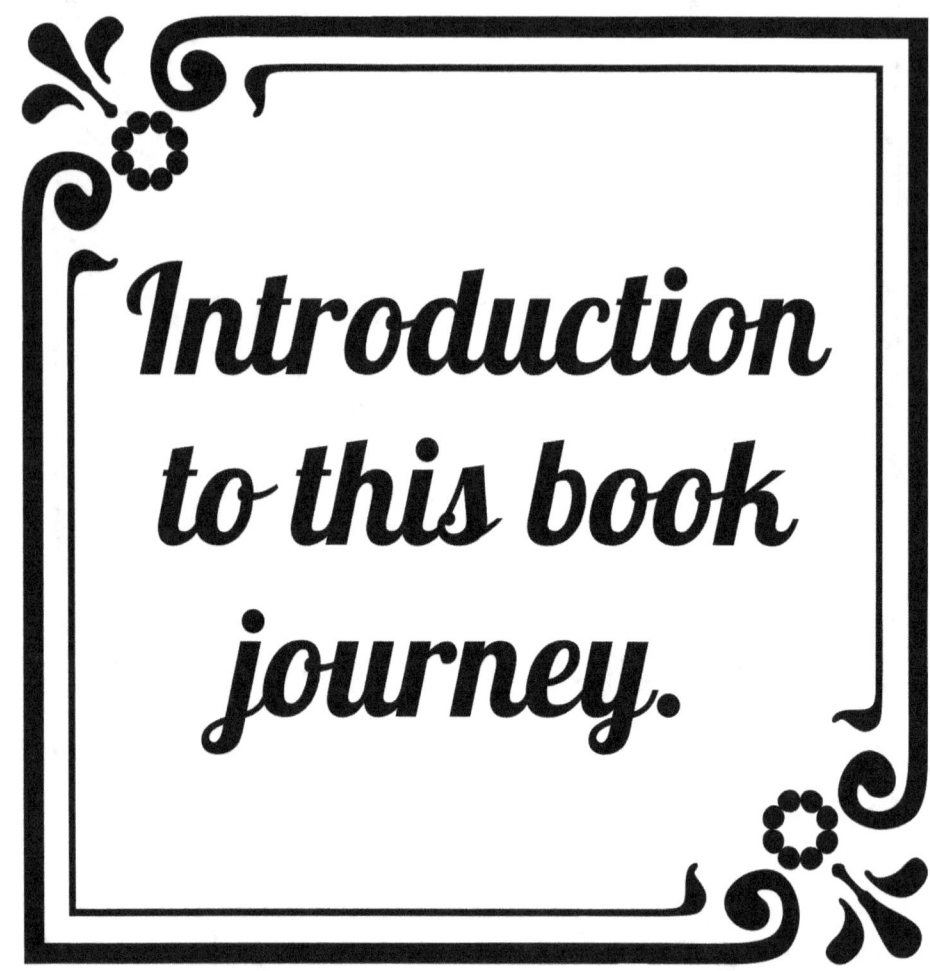

Introduction to this book journey.

I wrote "healing while hurting" in 2020. A book of poetry and reflections around the journey of grief when my dad transitioned. I remember when first thinking of everything the book would have in it. I wanted journaling pages, pictures, dedications, a thank you section, stories and more. I wanted it all.

Not everything made it into that book. Towards the end of 2022 I was feeling called to create a journal, to accompany healing while hurting.

I was already working on "Healing while writing" but it was going to be a book of poetry and reflections over my lifetime. ThenI decided, that title was meant for this book/journal. My first book was truly about me healing through writing.

Writing helped me in my time of grief. So did the pain. But it feels like it all makes sense, that it was supposed to be this way.
I decided this is how I will honor my father's next anniversary January 21, 2023.

Many people have shared so much with me about my first book and it just feels so right that this would be what's next for my author journey.
2022 has brought me back here, back to my dad- back to my first book- back to where "it started." At least this self-publishing journey part of my life.

Grief has come in many forms and situations and layers. This journal is for grief. Yes to "accompany" healing while hurting, but also to just be in partnership with grief in general.
My hope is you participate in writing in hopes of it helping with the healing journey.

Healing while Writing

is truly what "healing while hurting" is. Different titles and for good reasons but what got me here was writing. What got me here was what was created from the hurt, the grief, and the gratitude.

So much poetry and reflections and stories were documented and created. Healing while writing is for you. For the writers, the people- who need another way to cope and release.

I share my original Facebook posts and journal pages, yes with typos and errors.
I share this way on purpose with a purpose. I choose not to have an editor change anything.
I want to share in this real way.
I feel like this way of being, of my being- is a part of my purpose here on earth.

My reason why, for all of this- for this book- is because I am listening to my heart. I am practicing living in my truth, following my dreams even when the fears scream. I want to be transparent and open- in hope that others will feel it is ok for them to do the same.
This journal is yours, however, you choose to engage with it. No judgment!

What is your heart calling you to?

3/3/22

Allow the miracles to happen

I would not say, nor do I believe that my dad's passing and journey was for the purpose of me to write a book.

I do believe that miracles happen and can't be planned.

I never would have thought, my journey through grief and healing of losing him would turn into my first book.

I remember writing his obituary and saying I could write books and newspapers about him. I meant it. But, never did I really think it would be what it is.

This journey not only became my first ever self-published book. But it has been way bigger than that. It has become me living a dream, my dad living on beyond his life here, me living in my purpose, our family living beyond time itself.

This journey has done so much for my family. Helped us pay bills. Helped us dream again and know we are limitless. It's created opportunities and connections and so much more.

Who knew, this would all come to be?
GOD knew, even before me.
even though it was within me the whole time.

Had I known, before- it probably wouldn't be what it is.
It is what it is, because of timing. Because of what's meant to be.
and it's just the beginning. There's so much more coming. whether I know what it is or isn't. I can feel it

I've been on this healing journey, my whole life.
We just reach different chapters of it.
But this journey has been forever.

some of us reach these parts of ourselves with yoga, meditation, support groups and what not. And we tend to hear language like "how long have you been on your healing journey?" or "it looks like you are on your spiritual path."
and sure, that's true.
but I have always felt a little off with that statement.
Because truth is, this healing and spiritual journey has been forever. My whole life, I am sure.
It has just looked different at different stages.
and sometimes we don't have the language or perspectives or experiences that we do at other points in life.

but much like the journey of grief.
what I know to be true, especially with illness like cancer. Grief starts even when the person is alive.
and we can go deeper than that. we can go pre-diagnosis and still have some grief in certain relationships and life.

So truly, the grief journey is no timeframe.
we just have "time-frames" of different chapters.
but the journey. well, for me. Feels like it's always a part of me.

This is my invitation to you, to acknowledge and celebrate yourself.
For your journey.
with grief.
with healing.
with both or anything or everything else.
Your journey is beautiful and powerful because it is yours.
and you are a gift to this world.

Whatever part of your journey you are on. I hope you feel seen, valued, and whole.
Because, we are always whole- as we are.
and you are always "on time."

GRIEF AND GRATITUDE

Gratitude moves me along,
Grieving will help me move on.
Does not mean grieving ever stops
It just means feeling your feelings brings a
type of healing, that gratitude alone does
not.
It means gratitude helps me find grace
On those hard days where anger takes place.
In the moments of wanting to give up
Gratitude saves me, supports me in holding
on.

Allowing myself to intentionally grieve
Is what I'm learning I now need.
Because so much has shifted and
transitioned this year
And instead of breaking down, I didn't allow
being broken to be here.
I just kept moving along with the broken
pieces

Wondering what would break me
I just kept accepting the transitions
Never feeling whole with each piece, I lost of me.
Grief and gratitude can be in partnership
I need to allow each to be fully present.
November 23, 2022

1/30/18

4 years ago we laid you to rest. It's still hard for me to think of that day. It was absolutely beautiful considering the reason why.

We don't visit the cemetery too much, but we will again sometime soon.

4years ago was such a hard painful challenging beautiful day.

Miss you always dad.

Still grateful to all who came out that day

Lena Ayala-Velasquez 1/20/20

Shared with Your friends and Juan's friends.

6 years ago, was a heartbreaking day. It was the day I had to face the reality I never wanted to face. The reality is that I would lose my dad. That I would have to say goodbye.

and still, part of me thought I could save him. that my love for him was so strong that GOD would heal him. That he changed his life for the better so much and this wasn't going to be the end.

Just days before we had gone on a trip to Sonora, he was supposed to attend but he didn't. He had too many liters drained from him, he was tired, and he needed rest. This was the last opportunity for the Sonora house. We thought of not going. He wanted us to go, he wanted us to be able to take that last trip to that house. I wanted him there.

Part of me wanted to force him to go because I could see the end could be near but I didn't want to believe that. the other part of me felt he needed rest with us all out of the house. we didn't speak of his cancer; he didn't want or like it on social media–or even to be brought up in daily life. He wanted to live as if it wasn't there.

He wanted to just be seen for himself, not his sickness. so, we mostly kept to that. Living life making the best of it. I'm sure some part of him wanted us to stay, only he knew his true feelings. I feel horrible I didn't stay; I feel horrible I wasn't there those two days because that's two more days we could have had. I feel bad I didn't convince him to come–to see that view and place and be with us. If I knew his final days were really in front of us–it would have been different.

6 years ago, I went to the room and asked if he wanted to come to eat with us. He said no. I should have known. maybe I didn't want to know. he would always get up to go with us and say "when I can't I won't." he wasn't speaking much.

I thought he needed more rest. he was tired. he was drained. so, I tucked him in because I dint want him cold. I was going just a few blocks away and not for long-told him I would bring him back food.

I remember feeling helpless. all these years later I wish I stayed but everything happens for a reason.
at lunch, my mom calls and says my dad won't wake up when I say I dropped everything, I mean literally. I dropped everything. those babies I love so much, I left them with their dad who was working and family who were with us. I ran the fastest ever, beating the sounds of the ambulance and firefighters.

I am screaming to the sky "don't take my dad , dad don't leave me."

I made it home to see him on the ground. I was talking to him but he wasn't responding-just looking at me. they give him a shot to help his blood sugar and it seems to help. I feel so bad if I hurt him by asking him to please not leave me-knowing he was tired and probably ready.
I wasn't hearing any good news. and this was one of the longest days ever of watching him get put through so much. two different hospitals. I remember telling the doctors "keep him alive, keep him here with me." his wishes were written "let nature run its course."

I couldn't ride in the ambulance because he was in critical condition. I was being asked about his wishes in case he stops breathing. sitting in ICU for what felt like forever.

To me, he was getting better. he was awake, trying to talk, trying to move the doctors away........ I just knew he was going to get better... but the night was long.

one of those days and nights and situations where it's not where you'd ever want to be and yet there's no place you'd rather be.
these feelings hit me strongly still. I can still smell the hospital, the blood. I can still feel the emotions. I still question my choices.

oh how I miss you, Juan Ayala

is it hard to be thankful at times like this? sometimes. but I was thankful to have that time, family support, and opportunity to accept the journey for what it was and to be a part of it. I am thankful that years later I still am reminded I am human and I am not ok. it is ok to not be ok. and it is ok to be ok.
it was hard to learn that it's ok to be ok.

1/20/20

So much of today kept my dad's spirit alive and kept him on our minds. so much of today was about him while not even being in the plans. i am thankful for all that did work out even the stuff that didnt. its only 4:22pm and so many blessings have appeared.

1/21/21

Lena Ayala-Velasquez shared a memory.
Shared with Your friends and Juan's friends

Juan Ayala
7 years today, and I do still feel this way
Praying for myself as it all hits me, finally
Today ....no angel, my husband has work,
"Healing while hurting" is available on Amazon, it's a pandemic, it's a school day,
And it's thankful Thursday
The emotions are rolling in
It all feels hard again
In this moment.

Looking back to 1/21/15:

1 year ago, today I had to be the strongest I could ever be while feeling the worst pain I have ever felt.

January 21,2014 at 12:40pm my father Juan Ayala told me he was done with the machines, he was ready to be taken off and end the battle with liver cancer

You could see the fear and sadness and pain in his eyes, you could hear the faith and certainty in his voice

On this day last year, we faced the day, the moment-we never wanted to come, the inevitable point in life

On that day I not only had to say goodbye but I had to see my children say goodbye with not understanding why or what it meant

This has easily been the hardest year ever

Of life without an important piece of my life, heart, and soul missing.

A year of firsts - holidays, birthdays, days without him.

A first year of the rest of what life will now be

Digital frames, blankets, altar, memories, t-shirts and such all-around for comfort, for remembrance

.... last year I made hundreds of shirts and passed them out in his memory.

Please

if you have one, put it on. Share his smile and stories with the world. Help me, help him touch lives and forever live on

If you don't have a shirt, raiders or A's will do

I'm in the process of making buttons

"Don't thank me, thank GOD" he'd say and id reply "i thank him every day for you".

I feel like, I should be "better" already

Like, at this point - the pain should be motivating me.

The healing should be able to have me smiling

But yet I'm waking up unable to get past the crying.

I feel like, it shouldn't be this hard still

The fact that I've been laying for hours in bed, on this day- 7 years later feels unreal.

I just wrote a book about grieving and healing

I just released a book today but yet I'm still dealing.

My story didn't end with the last page of that book

My healing wasn't finalized with the outcome of that book.

Waking up this morning reliving that day 7 years ago

Upset at myself for not planning for today better

I was ok with knowing today was coming, everything was accepted — until early morning hours.

The day can't look how I wish it could

It's too late to plan when it's here now and timing isn't "good"

I knew I couldn't expect knowing how I'd feel today

But honestly, I believed, I would be ok.

And, I am

But it's all hitting different.

It still hurts the same, like that day

I feel out of place.

So much feelings all at once

So many thoughts.

It's gonna take some time

.... even after all this time

Juan Ayala really, really missing you today

Lena Ayala-Velasquez 1/20/18

· Alameda ·   1/19/17

A day of plans turned into a day in house, laying around, being sad, and emotionally up and down.

I don't like days like today. But you can't help how you feel sometimes.

Sometimes you just have to feel what's real and let it play out.

We made it to nations, but I couldn't eat, it was hard to smile and now the day is gone and the night is soon to be over.

Spent all day being positive and now it's all wearing off and I'm running into the negative emotions

It's been a very hard day on too many levels.

I think of you daily and still cry often.
Couldn't help it today my husband bringing up Saturday. And I kept thinking I should've made you come to that Sonora trip with us even though you weren't feeling good. You didn't want us to miss out and I wanted you to know you were more important than that. Not many days later we lost you and I always wish you would've made it there with us.

Someone asked me about you last week and I just thought how could anyone not know you. How could anyone so close to me not have had the chance to meet you.
All anyone needs is one interaction with you, to know your heart. Your smile. Your humor. Your strength.

Man I miss you.
The kids caught me off guard and
tears caught me off guard
"mom,what's wrong?
Why are you crying?"
"Sometimes I get sad"
I miss you dad.

1/21/21

*How could you be out thinking of you and
not me
Knowing what days like today mean to me
Knowing how they affect me
Knowing from the past what might help me
Even if I said I didn't know what I would
want or need
You should know
Even when I don't*

*That's not fair of me to feel
Not fair of me to be, you have your own
things to heal
You aren't a mind reader
I had enough coaching to know I need to
be clearer
And I'm not sorry for my thoughts or
feelings
I'm just processing*

Knowing it's ok to not be ok
Is not making any of this ok
Knowing it's ok to be ok
Isn't making it better today

feeling angry, sad, so many things
Searching to find what I know isn't
Like I don't know how to be realistic
Searching to find what's clearly missing
Knowing I'm not talking to myself how I'd talk to someone else with these feelings

I'm just processing
Today is such a different feeling

I didn't know how hard and painful this would still be
I didn't expect such a reality
 But this is me
This is my journey
I have to feel through it
It's the only way through this
......
oh dad, I'm sorry I'm a mess
I thought I'd be "better" than this
I know, I know.... I don't have to be sorry and it's ok to be a mess
I know, I know... I will get through this, it's just some hard moments

Juan Ayala I guess I've been "holding it together "for awhile
Trying to pull myself together, it comes in waves .... I cry then smile.

Lena Ayala-Velasquez January 21, 2021

After about 4+ hours of hard crying, of very triggered emotions.... I have been feeling now: more at peace, more calm and "better."

This morning was hard.

I received messages I never expected and I would just break down.

I was easily angered, triggered because of the pain, I guess.

I tried to do as many "normal" things as I could, that I knew "usually" bring me happiness.... those things both did and didn't "work"....

I was easily distracted and not as involved. But I do believe everything played a part in helping support me today.

The emotions may still come in waves ...but, for the past 2 hours I have felt more "me".... to I even cooked something outside of my "usual"... tator tot casserole....with a side of bacon, Iris said "why are you making that? did grandpa like it?

" It wasn't something he asked for. But he did love when I cooked.
I have now been able to smile and laugh without breaking down like the majority of this morning.

Grief and Healing are very strong. So unexpected what you will feel and go through. I needed it all today though. For what it's been so far. I needed those tears, those feelings, those moments.

I feel like right now I can move on with the day, with less anger, less pain and more gratitude/love/happiness/peace and clarity.

Thankful Thursday was made for today.
Today makes 7 years since you "left" this earth. Your favorite number 7.

Looking forward to whatever this day has left in store for me.
Juan Ayala miss you dad. love you

Lena Ayala-Velasquez 1/21/22

Shared with Your friends and Juan's friends

Sometimes, even as you try to tell a new story and live a new way
that anger, sadness, anxiety and past is just triggers away.
something about those feelings I have been away from all day

it only took one set off, to set off the minefield and take what was away.
and the thing about me getting set off, then the its domino effect
one by one each person falls next.

explosions all around
calm, peace, understanding, and happiness can't be found.
Now, we all need our space
build up is all it takes.

I realize, it's been building up all day
trying to avoid this pain and outbreak.
but now it's here, and I just want to let it go
no one is to blame, no one hurts more than
another—all you know, is what you know.
all you can own is your role, yourself
all you can control, is you and no one else.

she screams "this day isn't just hard for you,
you know"
.........I know, and yet I've been taking it on as
my own.
and I never had to
I was coping too.
even though I thought I have been ok
even though it's been different today, for me-
than past "anniversary" days
I have been too myself, even while moving
"together"
and now I am reminded, to be present, to be
right here.

1/21/22

Kathy Munoz thank you for my first "Pandemic Poetry" purchase. signed and mailed.

you are my first official purchase thank you beyond thank you.

I was first in line when the post office opened

Thank you for helping make my day that much more special.

thank you for supporting my journey and drafts in all of their imperfections. you support me with so much love. I am thankful for your comments, messages, and your purchase.

It feels so wonderful to be supported. It feels so wonderful that someone is excited and wants more (I thought maybe no one would after the "hype" of the first was "over.")

Thank you for helping me remember my "why."

To keep writing, sharing, trying and doing.

Thank you for reminding me that this feels so good.

LENA AYALA-VELASQUEZ 1/21/22

Today is my dad's 8th anniversary of his transition.

& 1-year happy birthday of our first book "Healing while Hurting"

*I am thankful for waking up, to life.
To memories.
*This morning I am thankful for my husband getting out the "grandpa blanket" and fixing our bed
*I am thankful to wake up to my mom who spent the night. and who came in to check on me last night when I was in my tears. She doesn't know how to handle those moments "but I don't want to see you sad"
*I am thankful for the 10 amazon book reviews
*I am thankful for all who purchased healing while hurting.

*I am thankful for all who want to purchase ratchet grandma when it's ready in its final form
and for those who want the "rough draft" form

*I am thankful for those who are waiting to purchase pandemic poetry and reflections.
both the unrevised and the revised formation
I am thankful this morning I approved the revision, upload and am awaiting the complete approval within the next few days.

Lena Ayala-Velasquez 1/21/23

And that's how the day has gone...

It's dark now...

So much left undone.

Although not even 6 pm. It feels like the day is over because it is dark.

we only have 1 car, which doesn't fit us all.

we tried to go to nations for breakfast but couldn't find parking- even though we had a friend with an extra car.

we couldn't go to the cemetery due to lack of space and cars.

we ended up not walking to the beach to use the metal detector due to naps and it being so cold out.

but we did make impromptu choices. we did get nations pie.

my mom showed up.

we ended up picking up my daughter's friend and our nephew tonight while out getting pie and milk.

it was a cup of noodles- amazon prime movie night.

we watched two movies.

Beautiful boy"
and "our friend."
very sad movies.
that sometimes got to me but not in the way my usual self would be effective.
It's almost as if I am too tired and numb to feel at the level I usually do.
Two friends...well family-sent me texts today.
To just send love.
Those were the two times that got to me the most. especially the text in the evening.

she asked how I felt and all I felt was incomplete.
In so many ways.
In the way that I have no tears.
I feel so tired.
we can't do the plans I wished cause of the car.
I don't know how I feel besides incomplete.
we are all together but all on our own, with naps and bed and whatnot.

emotions hit me when I was ready for bed and felt I didn't do all I could have or should have done today.

started missing those nearby.

I could blame the day. I know it's all in my mind.

today just feels not real. like today isn't today.

started regretting all I didn't do. started feeling sad.

Trying to find extra reasons to do just the "normal" things we would usually do. Like, get pie.

going back and forth with my mind about not getting it would be ok cause it isn't his birthday or a reason to celebrate.

then also thinking, he is a reason, his honor, our book we made, what traditions mean to the kids- the fact that they asked and I had to snap out of whatever zone I was in and find myself again and get up and get out and make life happen.

1/21/23

Today almost feels unreal.
Like today isn't today.
Like I just don't want to feel.
This is kind of new for me.
and in some ways not.

When sharing a child and having to figure out times and arrangements to make things work— -we are no stranger to certain days and dates having to be celebrated at other dates and times.

Acceptance and flexibility doesn't mean it doesn't come with grief of what you wish a day could look like.
Today is different in the sense, we are all together. No need for having to figure out how to share our oldest or take off work or anything.
because today is Saturday and our weekend.

However, a week ago someone tried to steal our car and just yesterday it went into the shop.

so, any plans we had that involved driving - are limited now.

because the car we have left does not fit us all.

Did I think about just some of us going to the cemetery. To make sure we showed up today- even incomplete? yeah- I thought about it.

but it didn't feel good or right.

The car will probably be fixed in the next week.

we already have decorations for the cemetery.

so, I decided we will go when we all can go.

even when circumstances and decisions are made. even when you think you made peace with reality. sometimes feelings sneak back in like sadness, frustration, anger even.

Of course, I had ideas and plans of how today could go.
but, instead, we kind of treated it like any Saturday.
I did feel the need to be in bed extra today.
I felt a lack of motivation at times and then urges for motivation at others.
I felt the need to rest.
No tears today but I held a loved one who was in uncontrollable tears.
we acknowledged today for what it is and means.

night-time comes fast these days which makes the day feel over before it sometimes gets started.
the kids all took naps today, long naps.
just allowing everyone to be.
be with the date, the day, the time, the cold, the feelings, and the flow.

LENA AYALA-VELASQUEZ

January 21, 2023 at 10:41 PM
Shared with Your friends and Juan's friends

It has been a long 9 years.
But I have learned grief started way before the journey "after"
and I have learned this, time and time again.
with different people and different situations.

why don't we talk about grief more?
especially when illness like cancer or situations like comfort care and hospice are involved.
That grief process happens even when our loved ones are alive.
It can be over years or months or weeks or days.

The layers to grief, and how we experience them are all different.

The reality that happens once they leave this world in this way.
It all takes its toll and journey.

Not to mention the layers to relationships in general we have with loved ones before a diagnosis.
grief can be present and real even without an illness or diagnosis.

Allow yourself to feel and be real.
cause this journey is a big one.
sometimes feels complicated and hard to understand.
but who says you have to understand it?
just allow yourself to be present and to heal- in your own way.

JANUARY 21, 2023 AT 08:44 AM

Today, 2 years ago now was the release date of my first book
"Healing while hurting"
Working on book 6 (healing while writing.

A journal to accompany this one) n honor and memory of my father and loved ones.
In partnership with grief and gratitude
But for now, celebrating year two- of book one.

9 years today.
In some moments I feel ok.
Some moments feel like the pain will never go away.
Sometimes I still fight for my dreams,
When they try to tell me you are still here and I'm arguing back knowing it's not what it seems.

Once again, this day is here,
And I'm laying in bed- just wanting to stay here.
Once again, a bunch of ideas about how today should go,
And plans are already not going how I tried to plan for them to go.
Went to sleep without tears falling,

Even went to sleep before spending too much time scrolling.

Scrolling for hours through pictures and old posts,
Knowing I'd get lost in the media of all I've seen in hopes of finding something new knowing I won't.

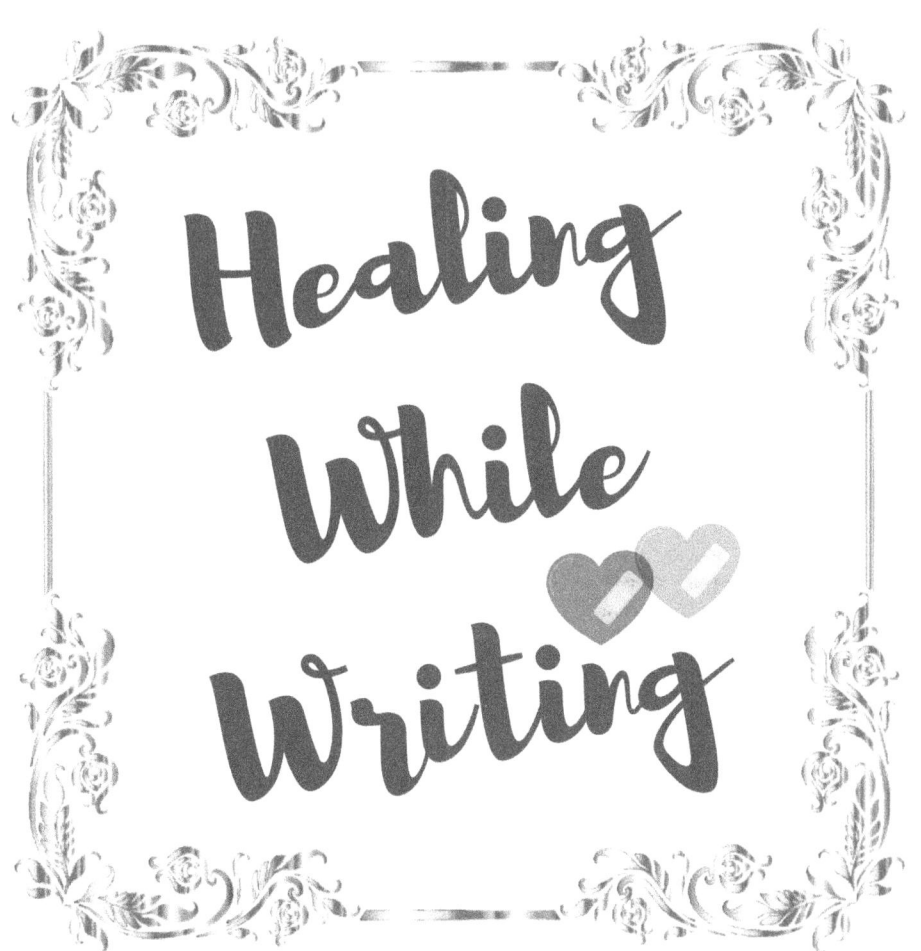

Healing While Writing

(Days, Weeks, Months, Years)

❄❄❄❄❄   ❄❄❄❄❄   ❄❄❄❄❄

The next chunk of pages is dedicated space for you if you want to reflect on the days or weeks or months or years about a certain person passing or to reflect on grief in this way. Sometimes numbers of days, dates and things in that nature might matter so much to someone when reflecting. (Example: Day1)

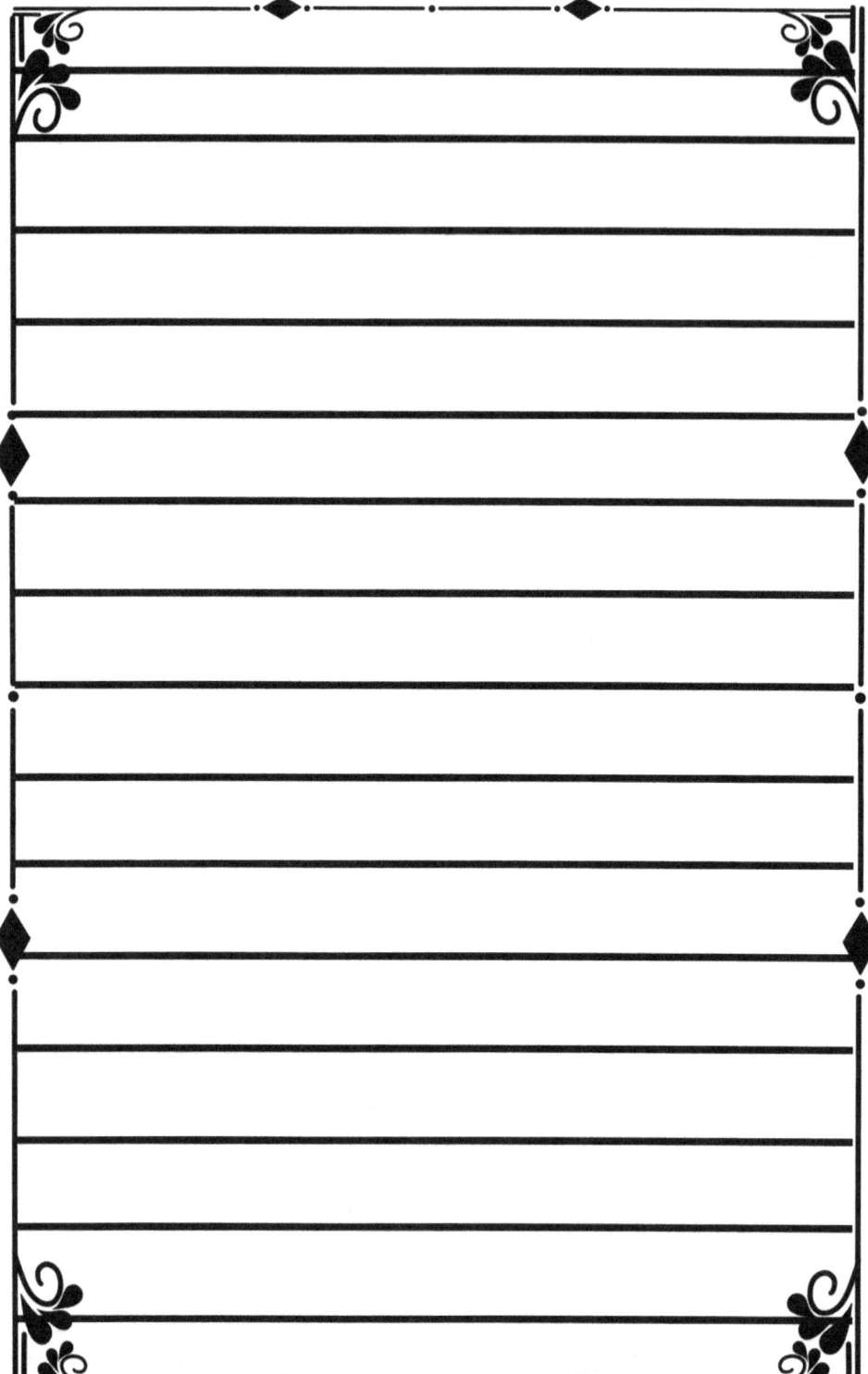

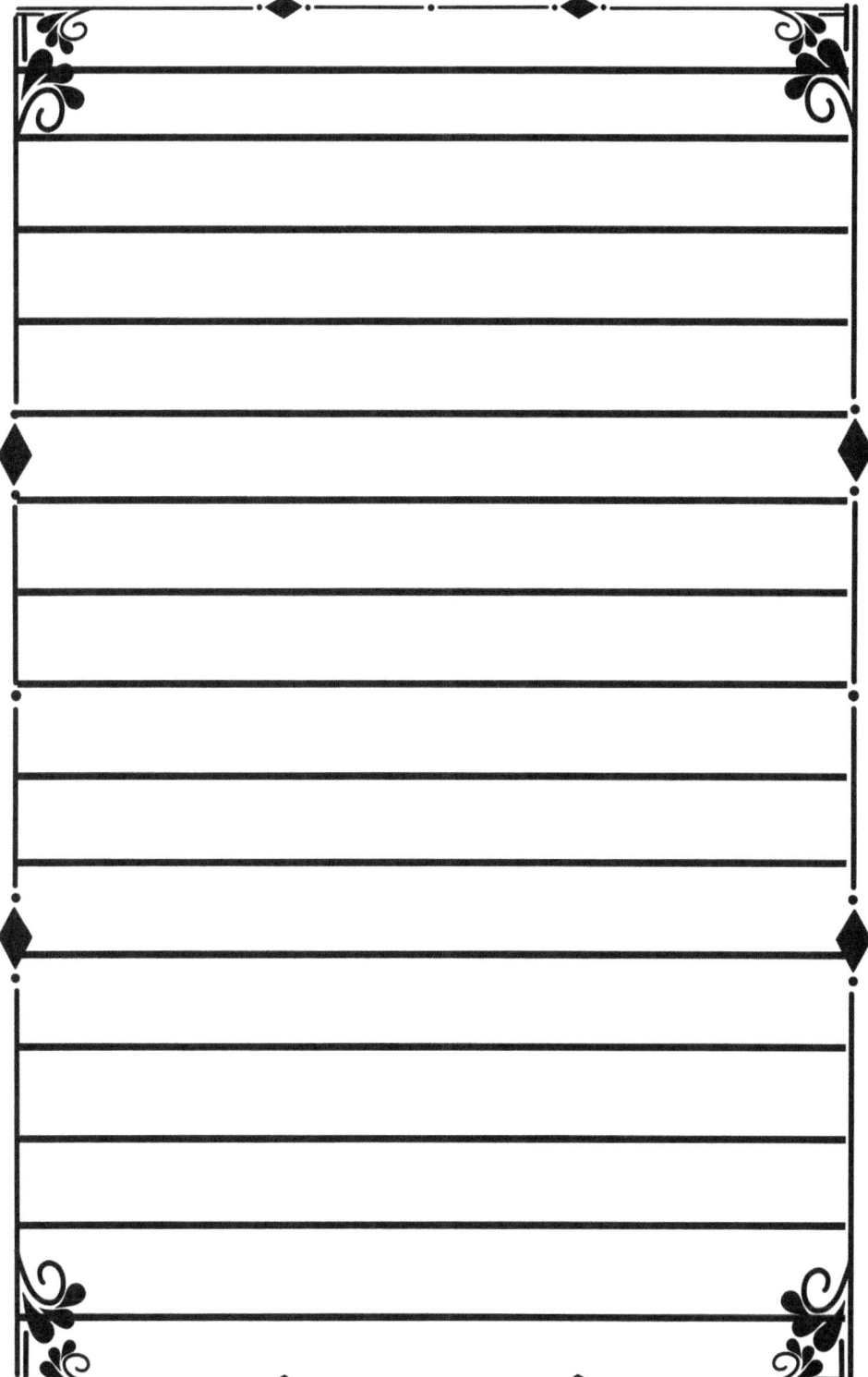

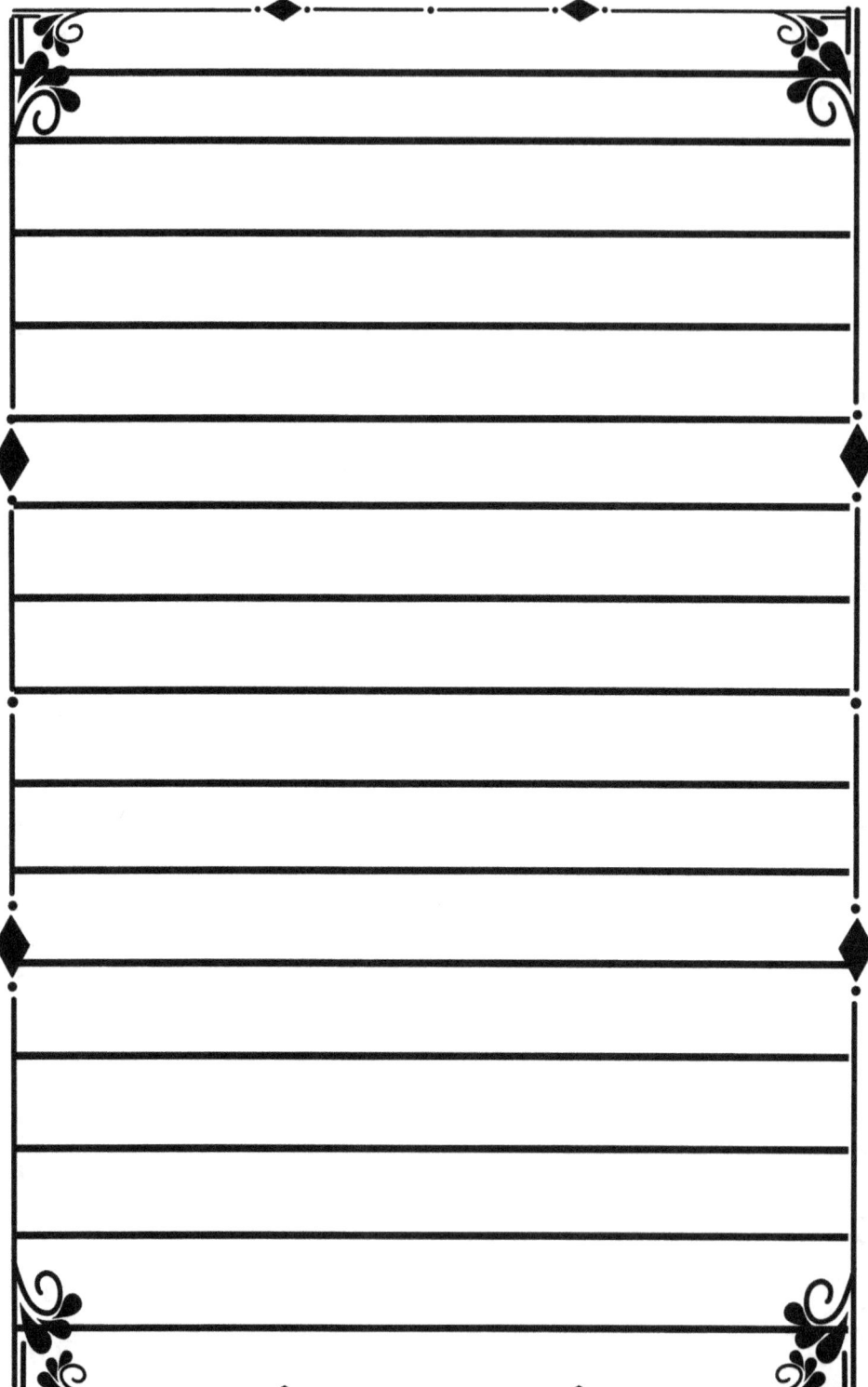

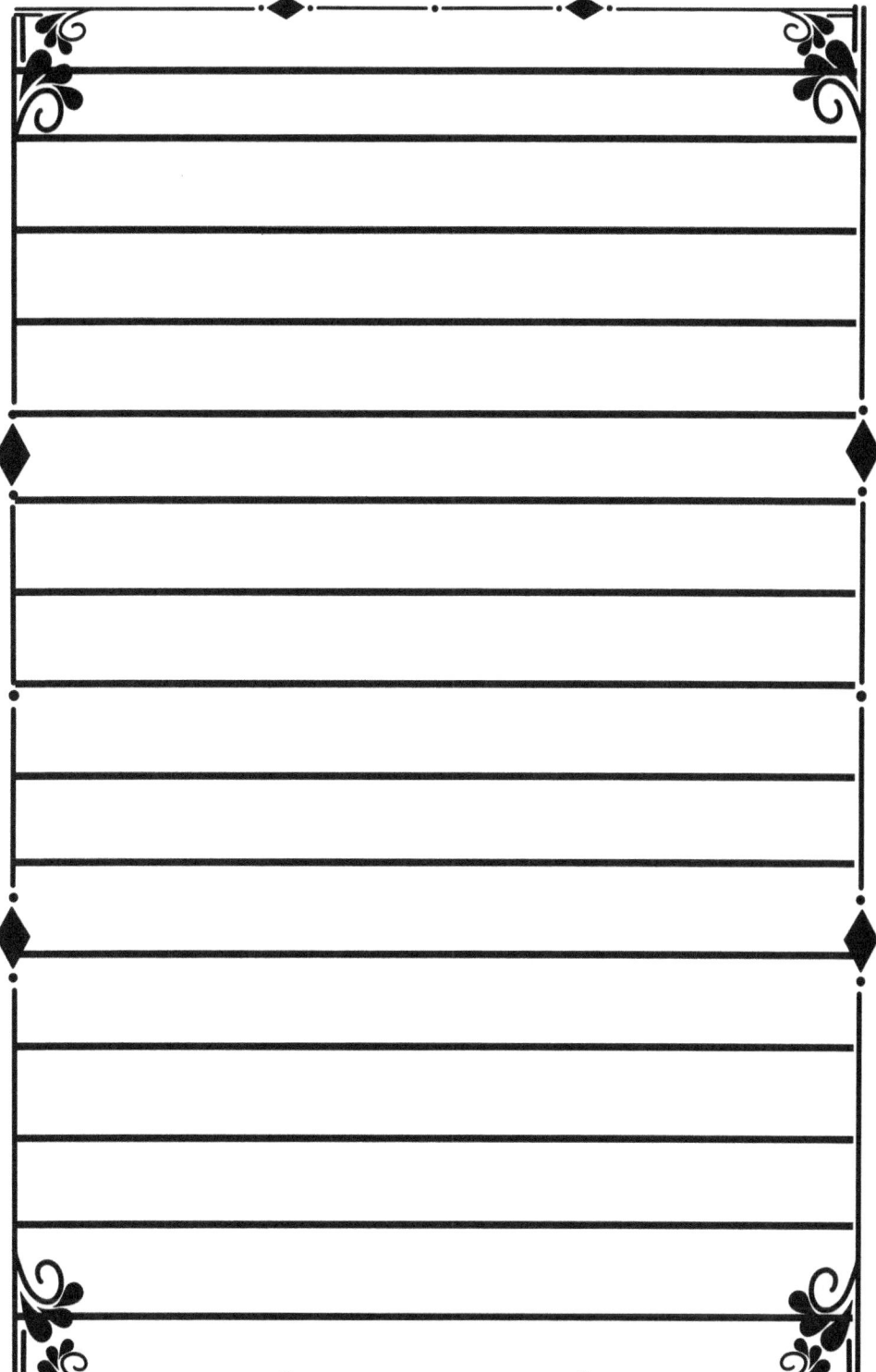

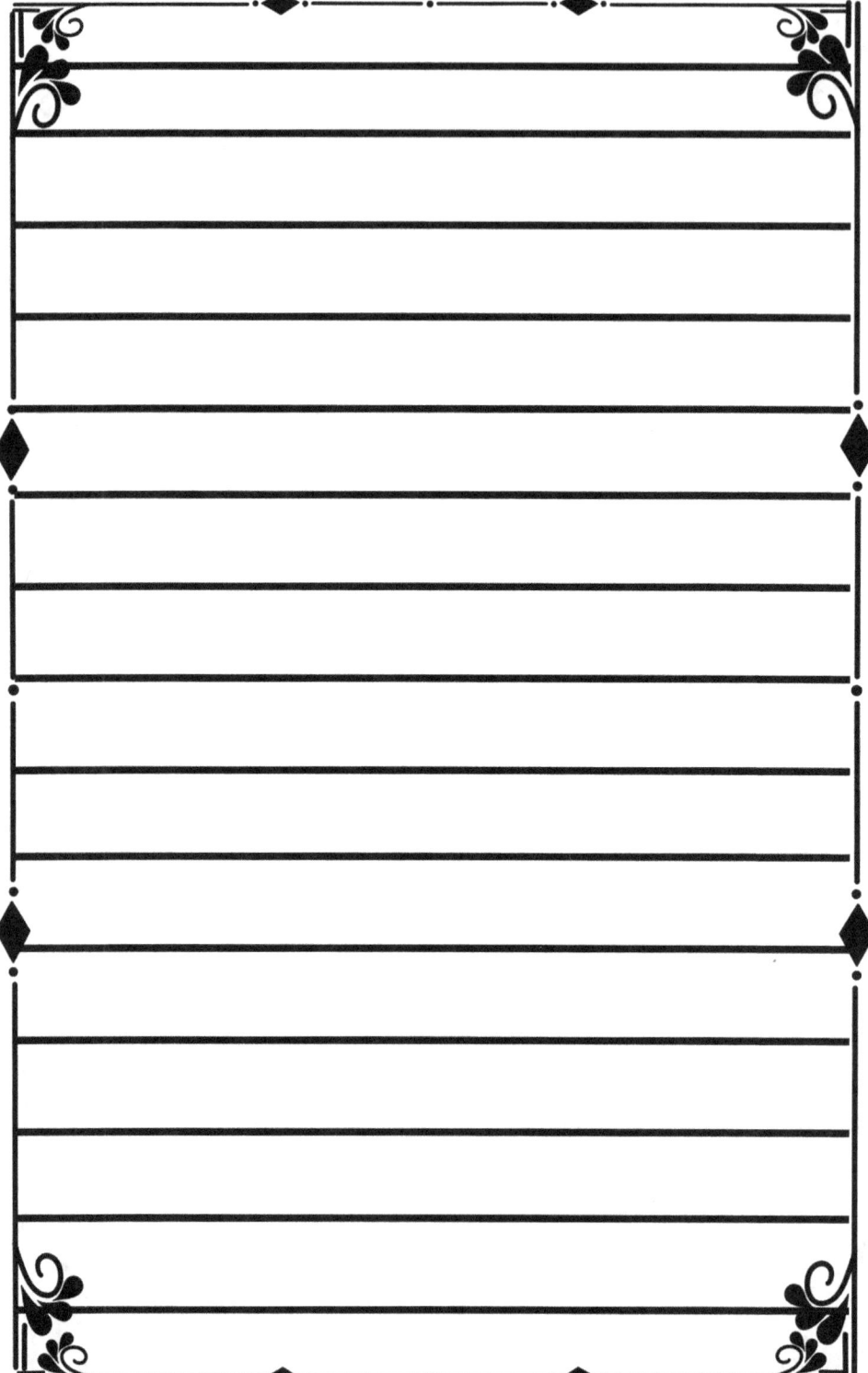

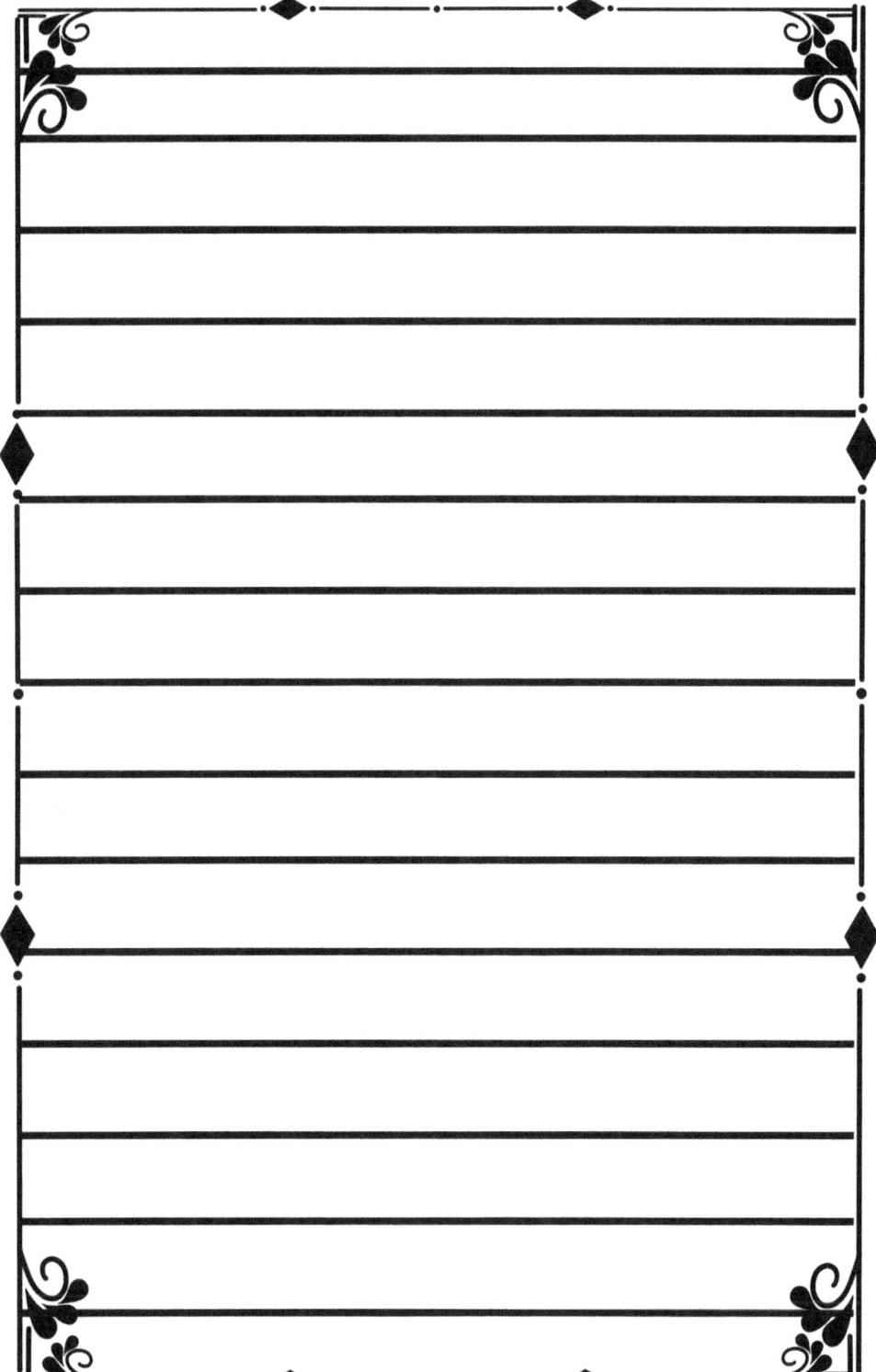

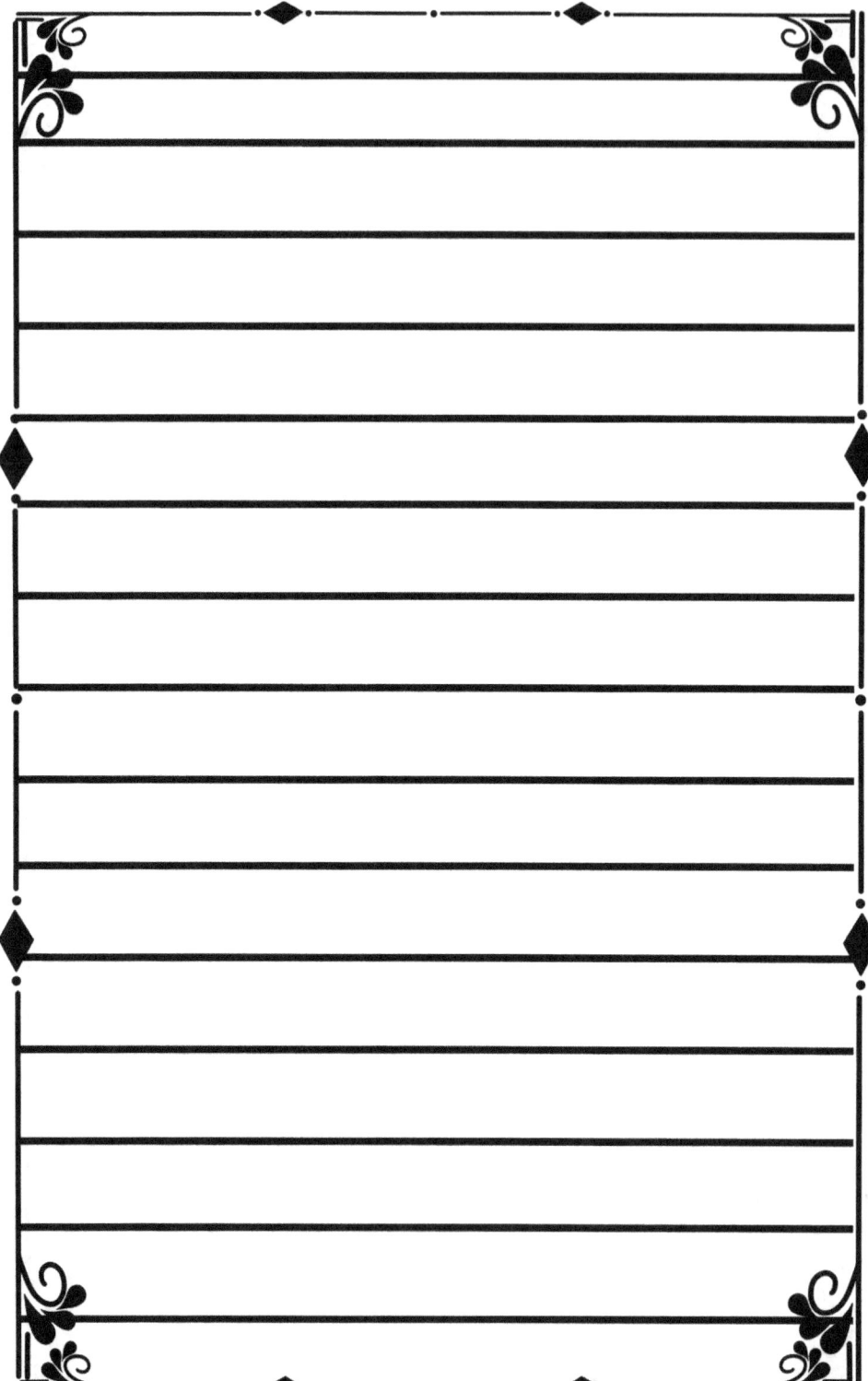

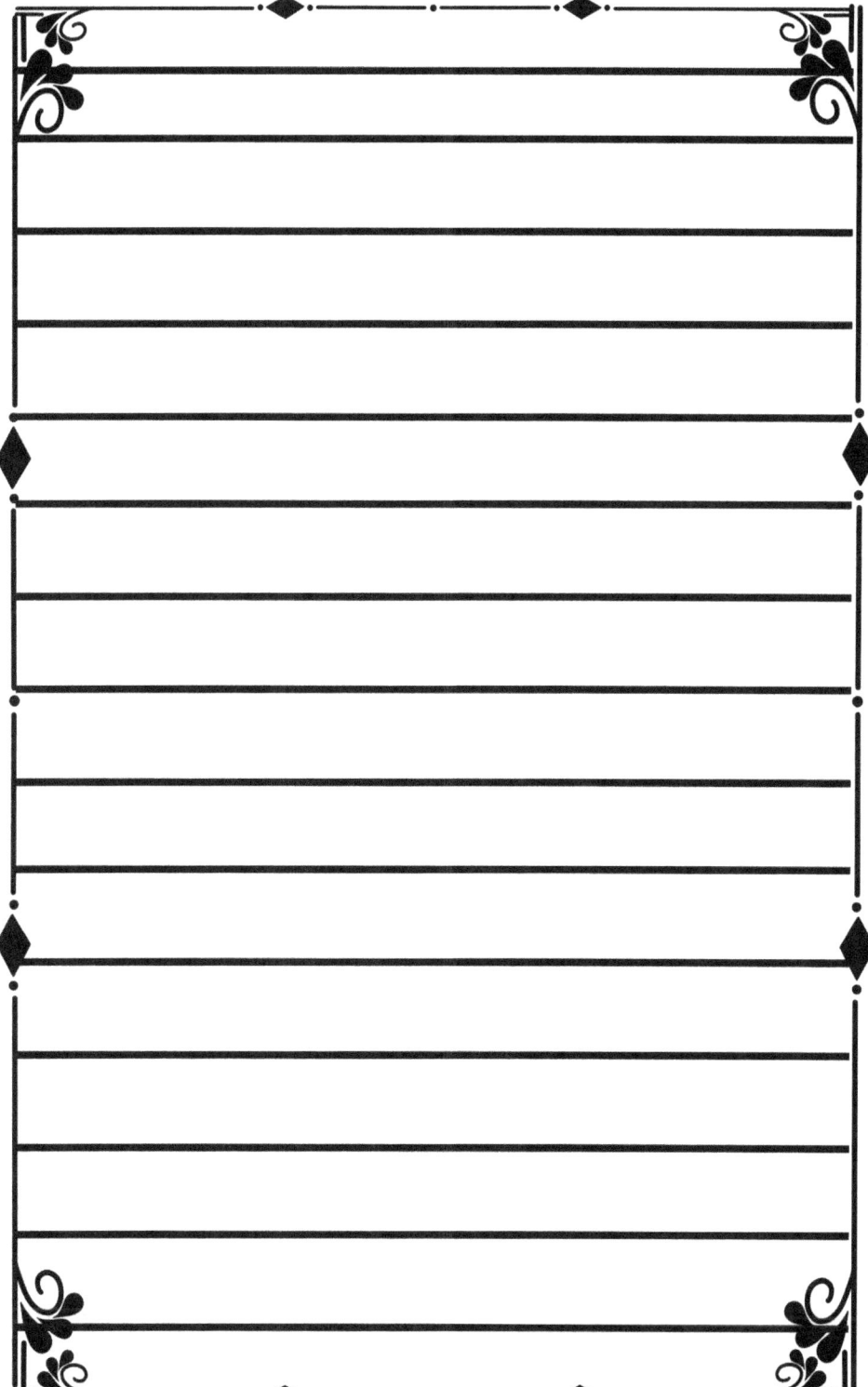

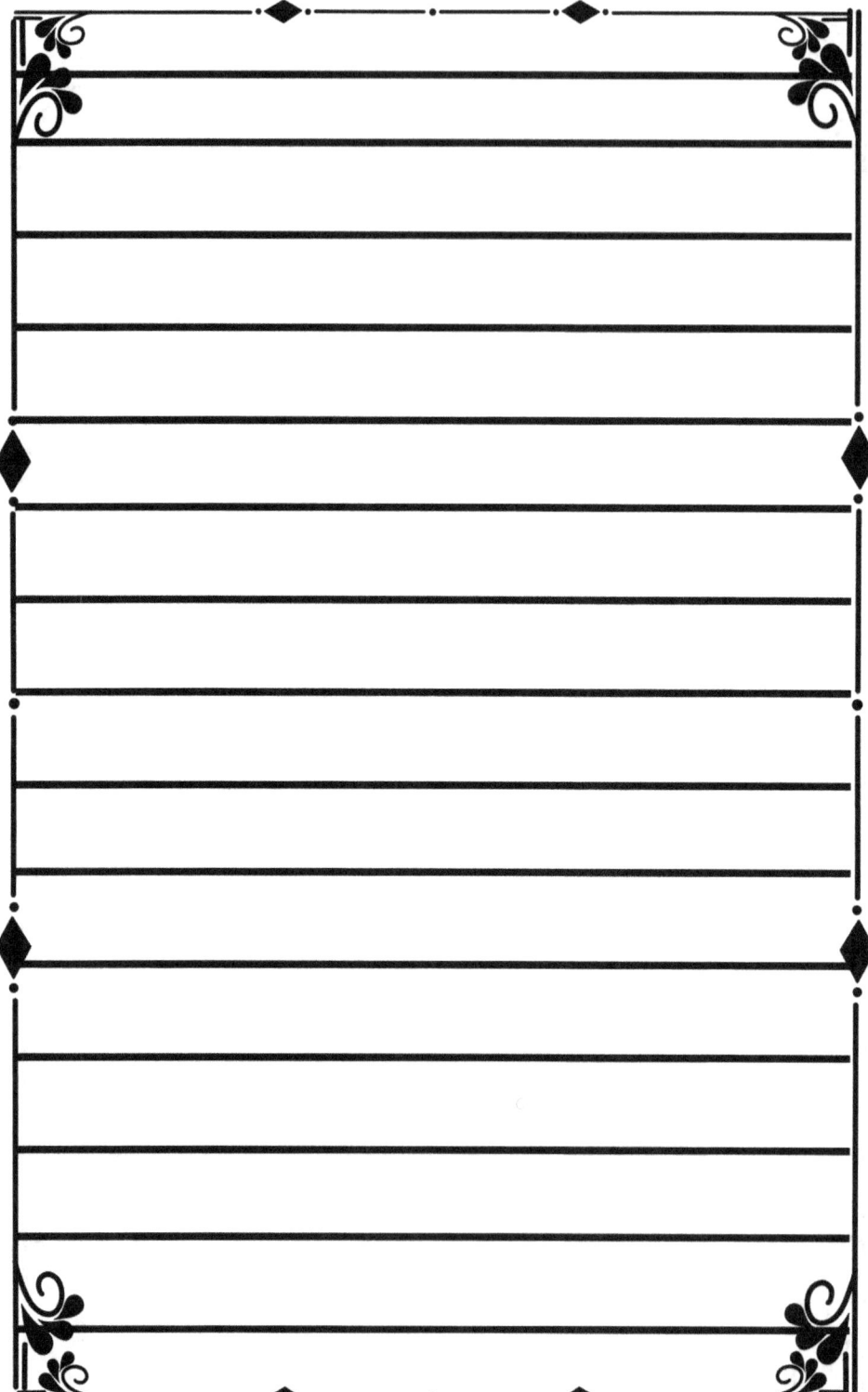

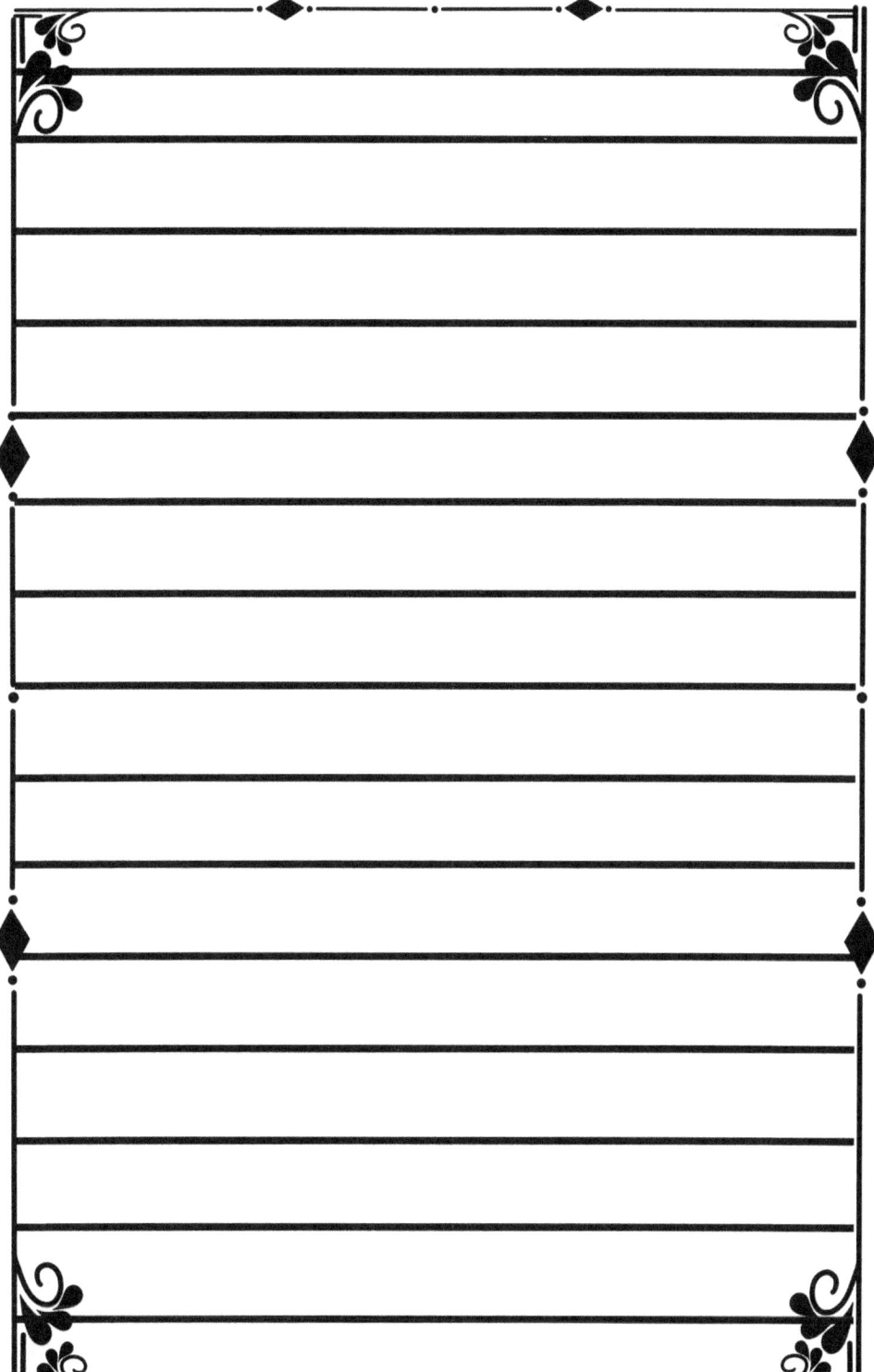

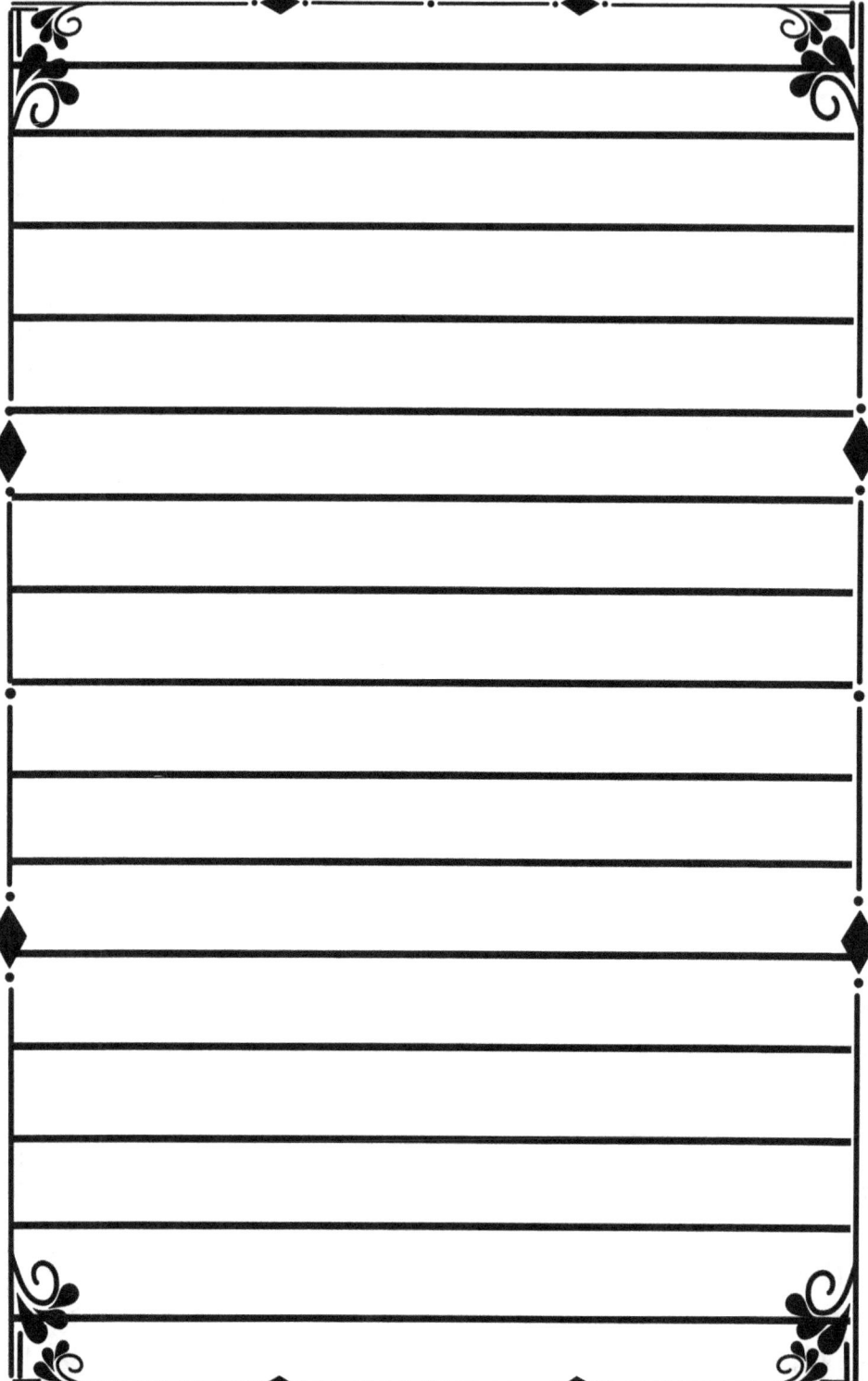

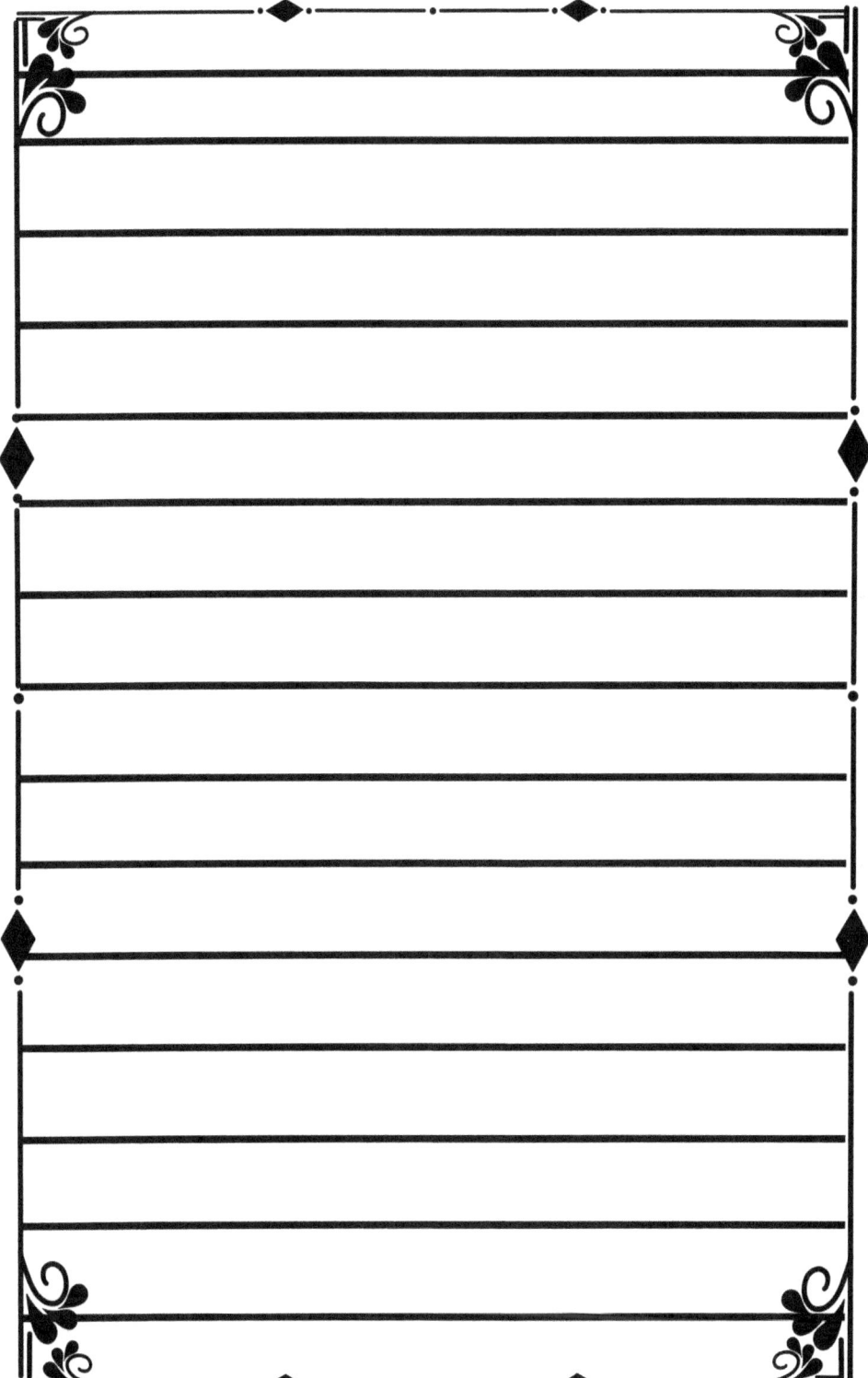

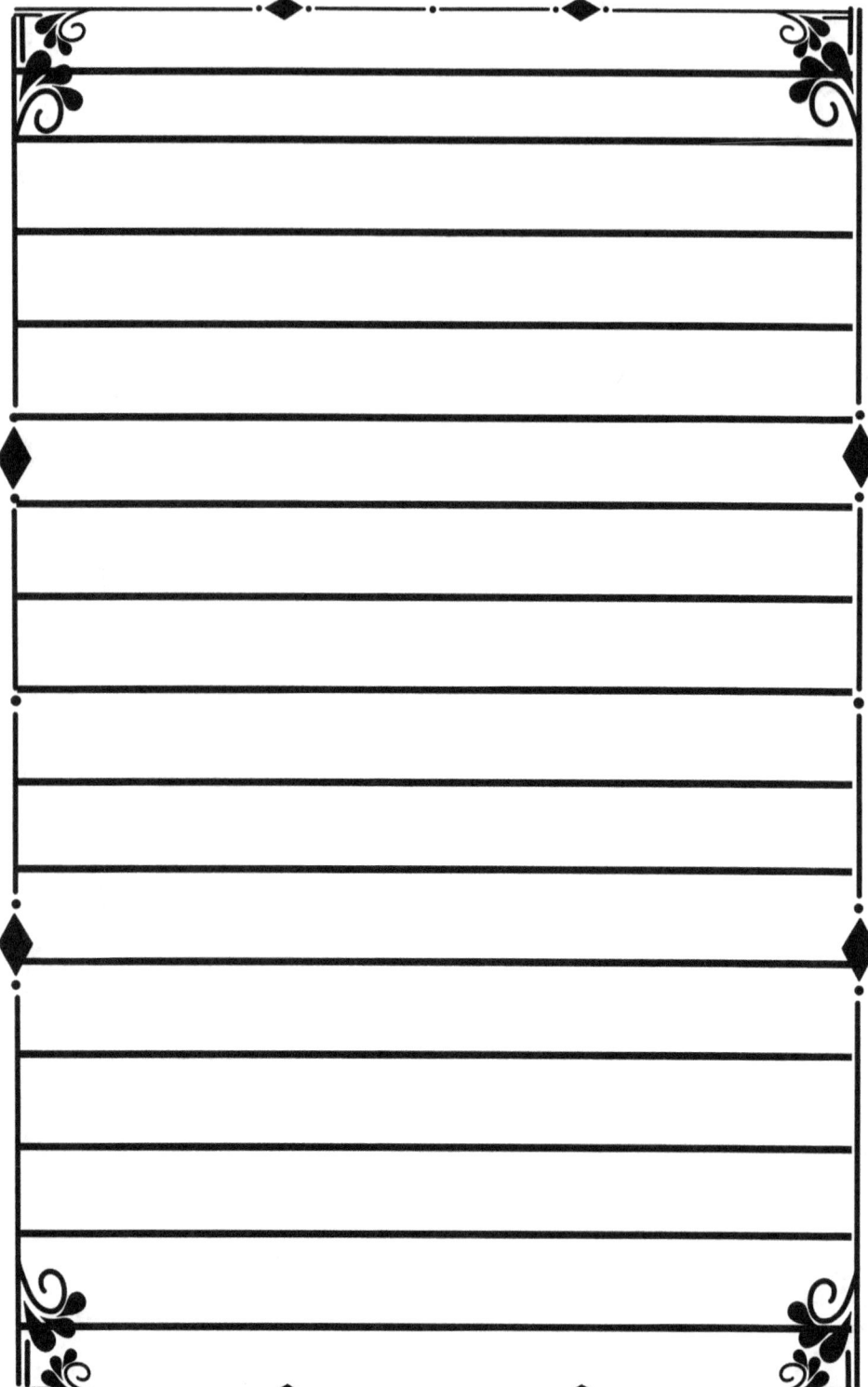

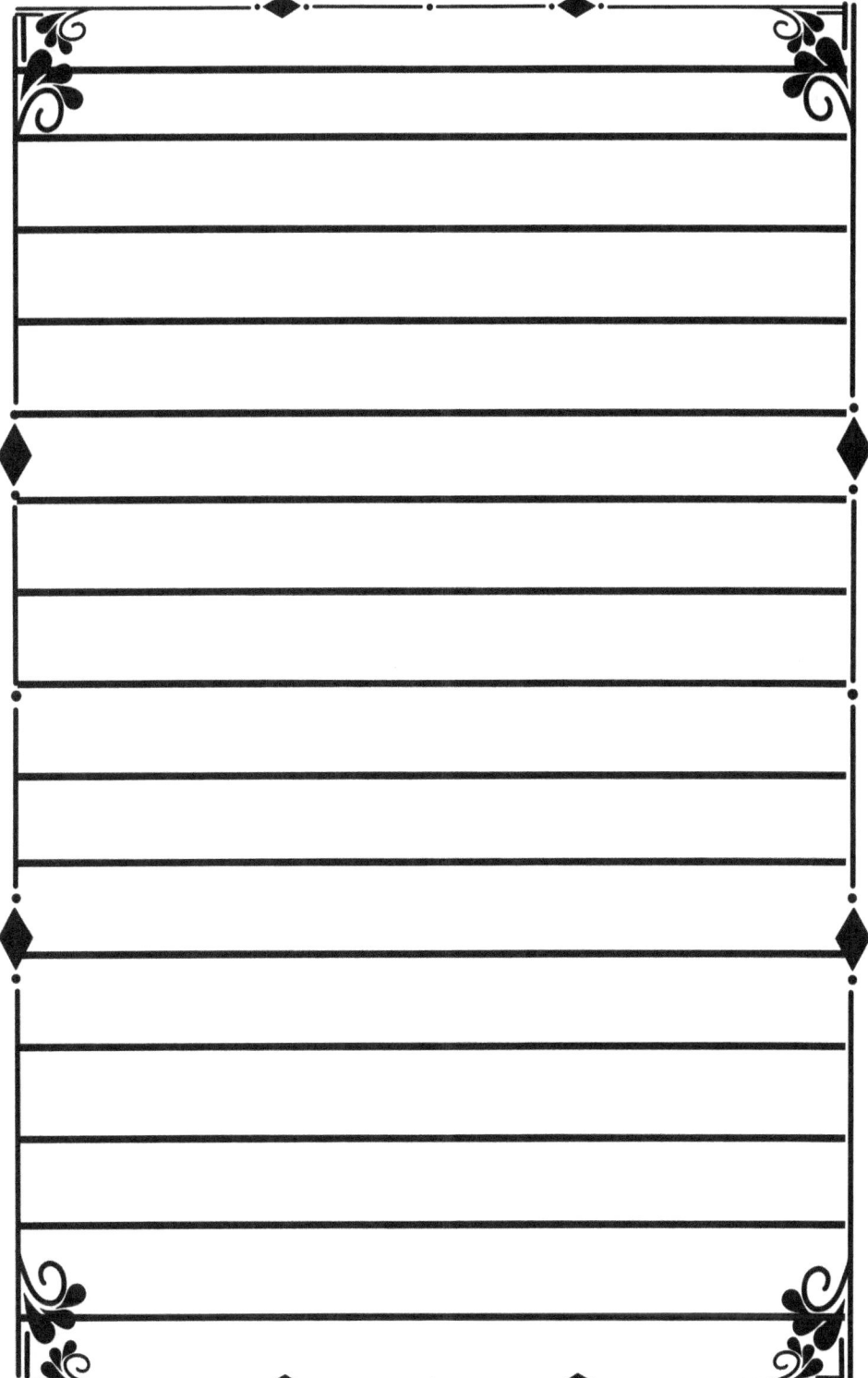

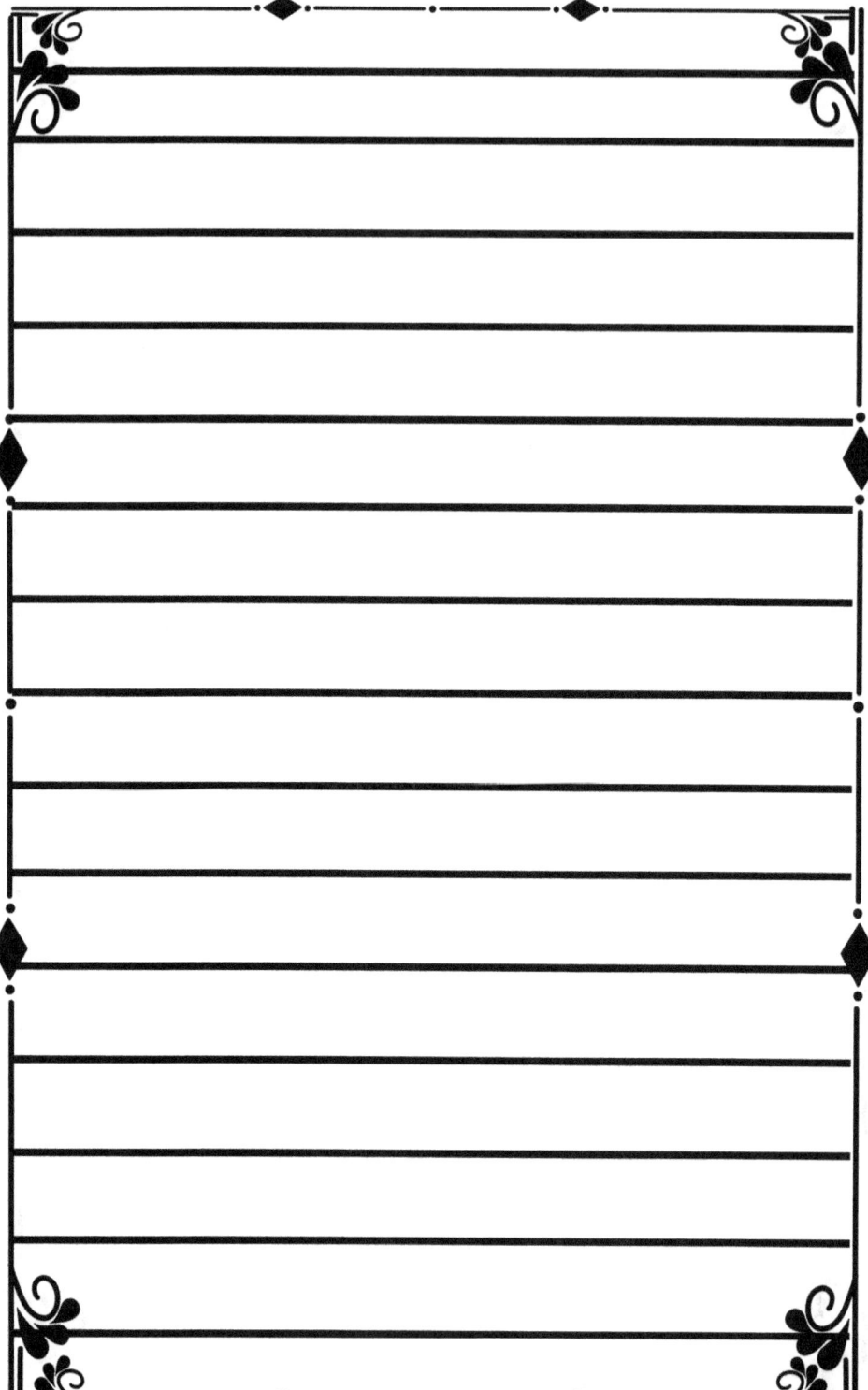

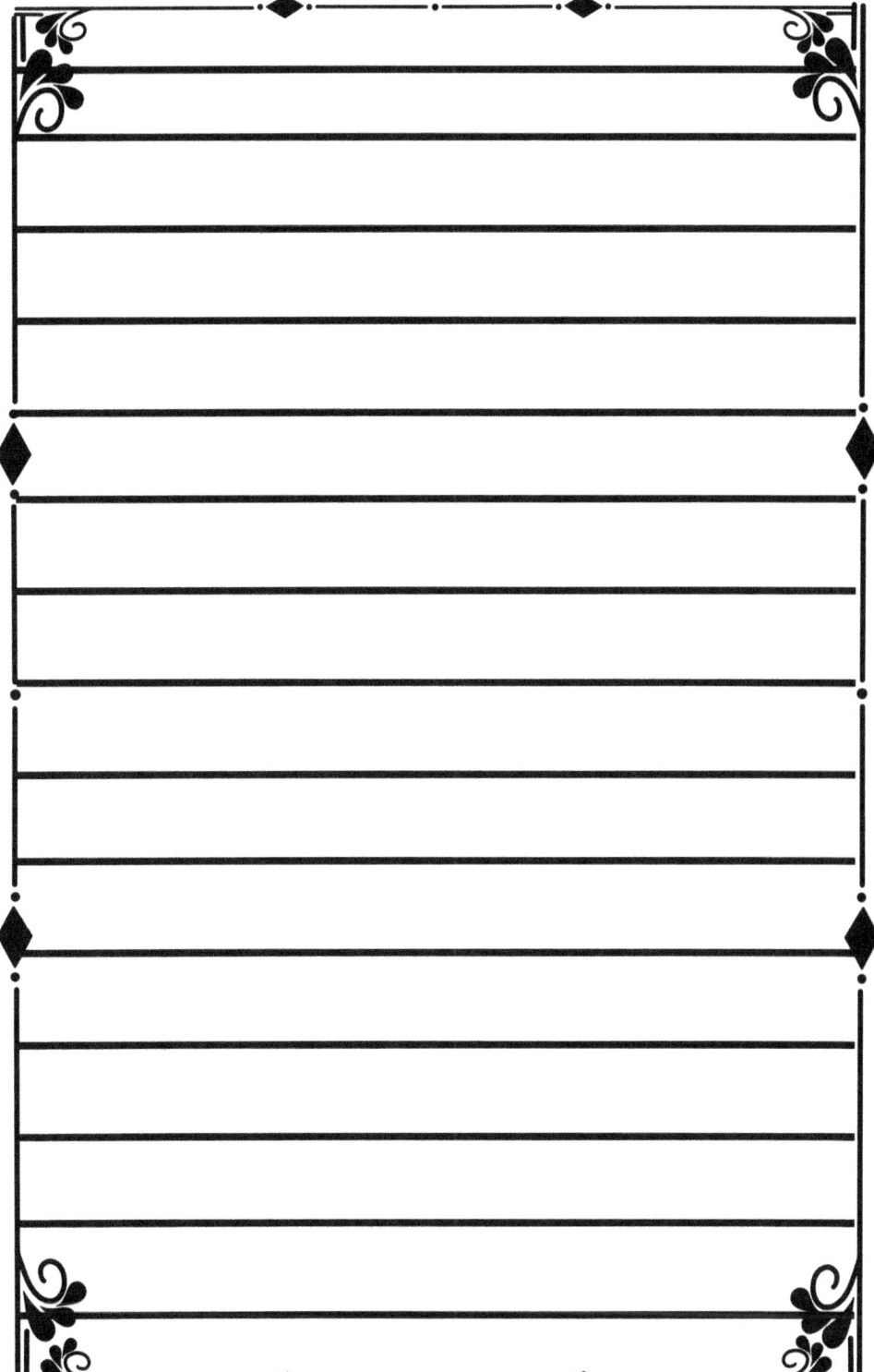

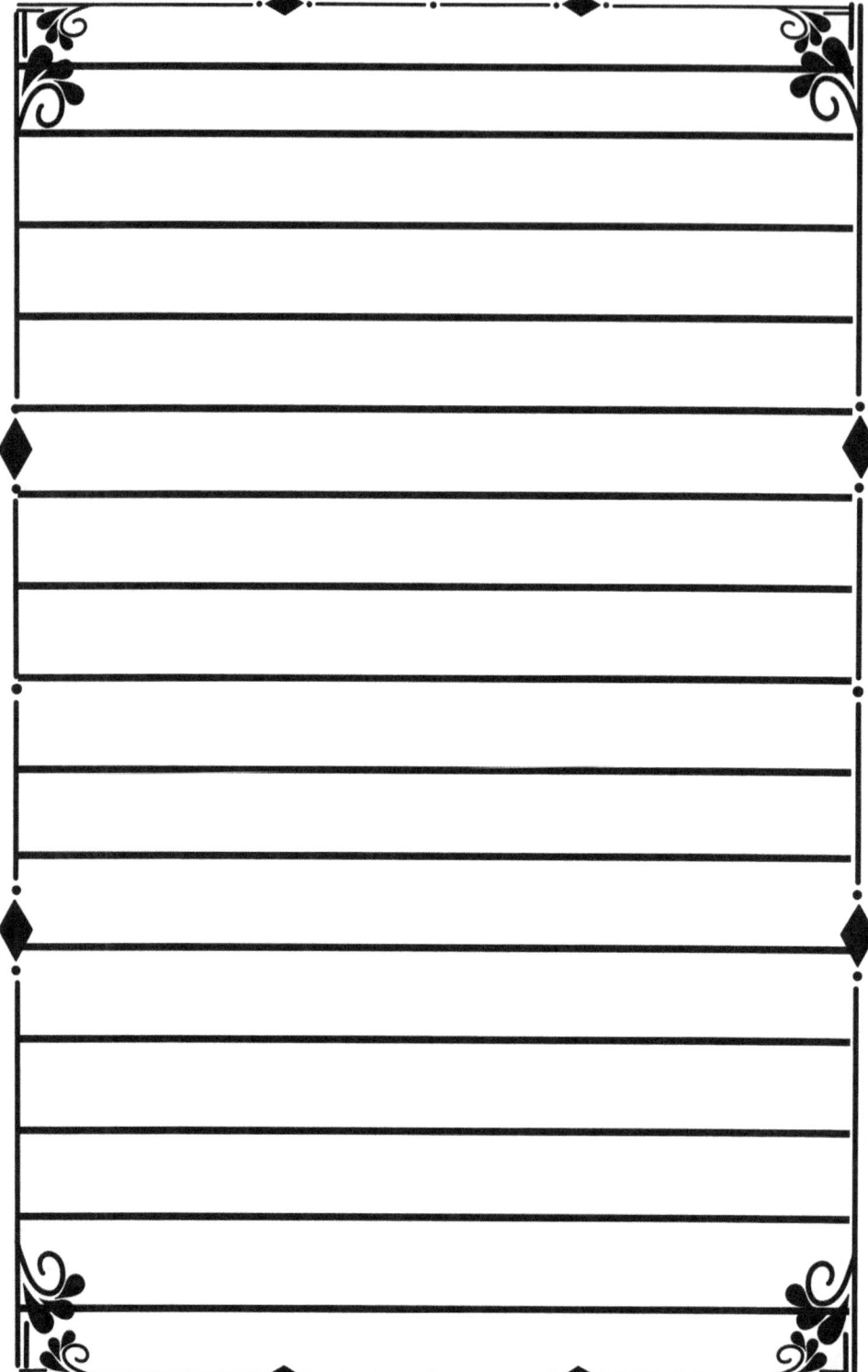

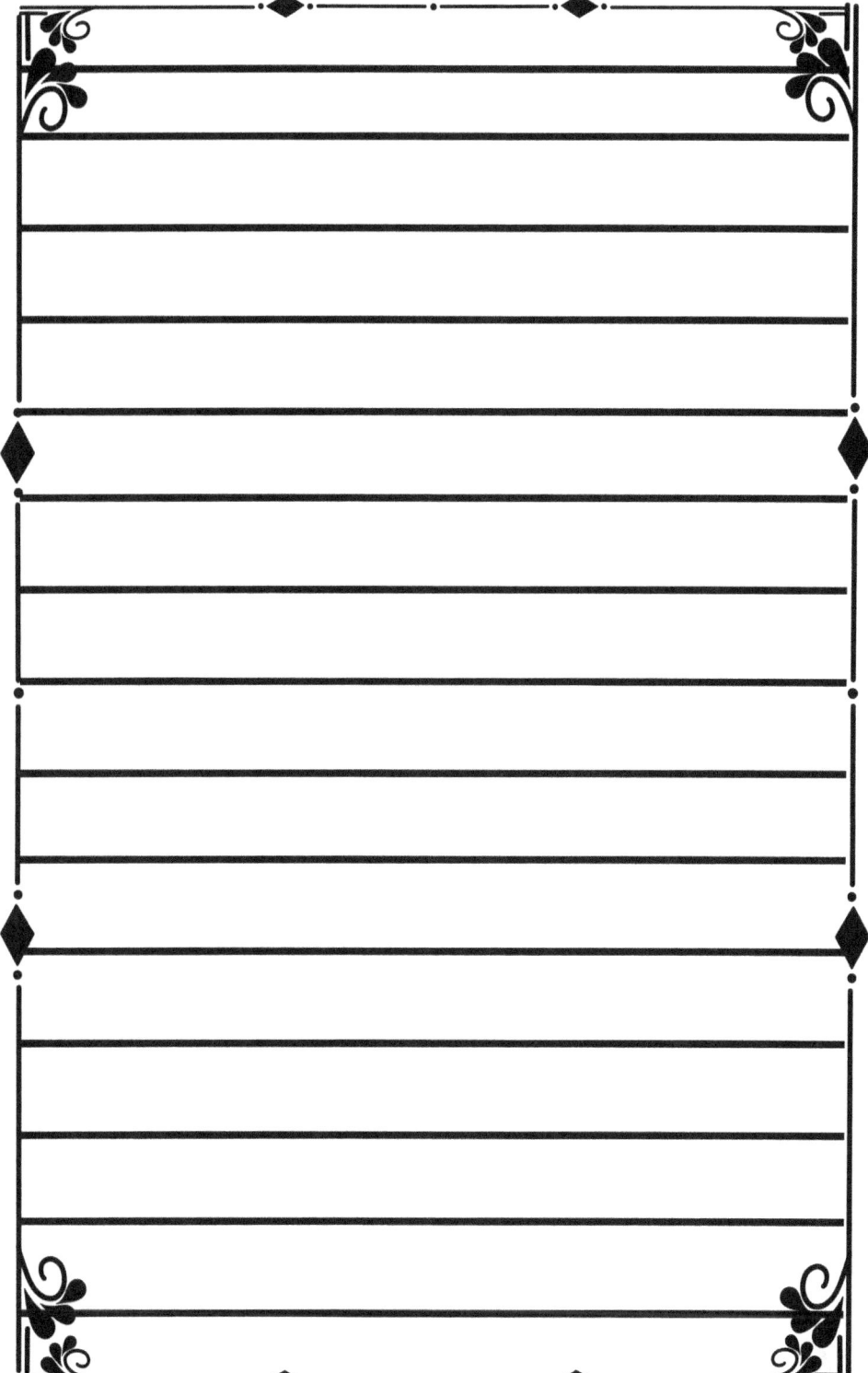

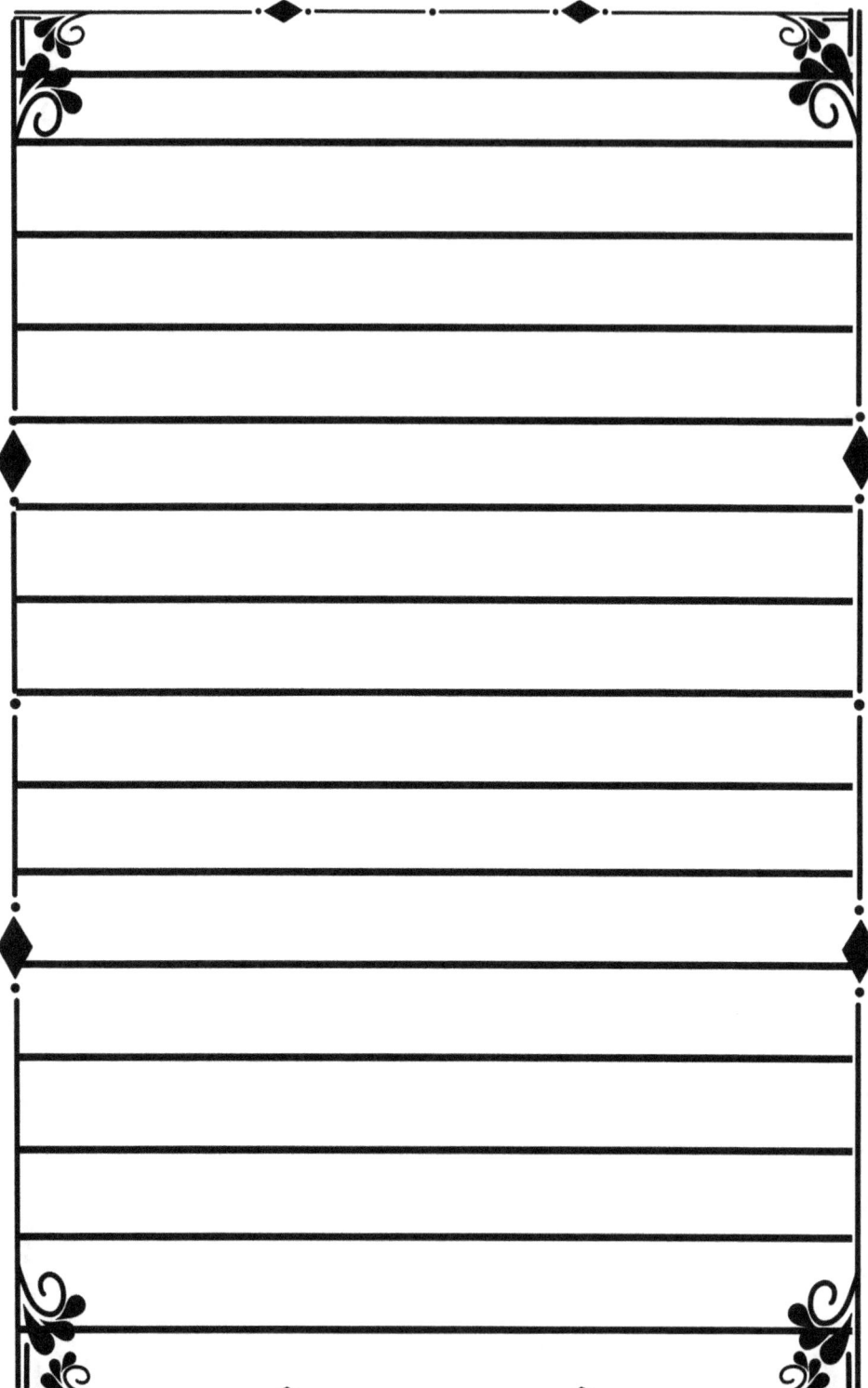

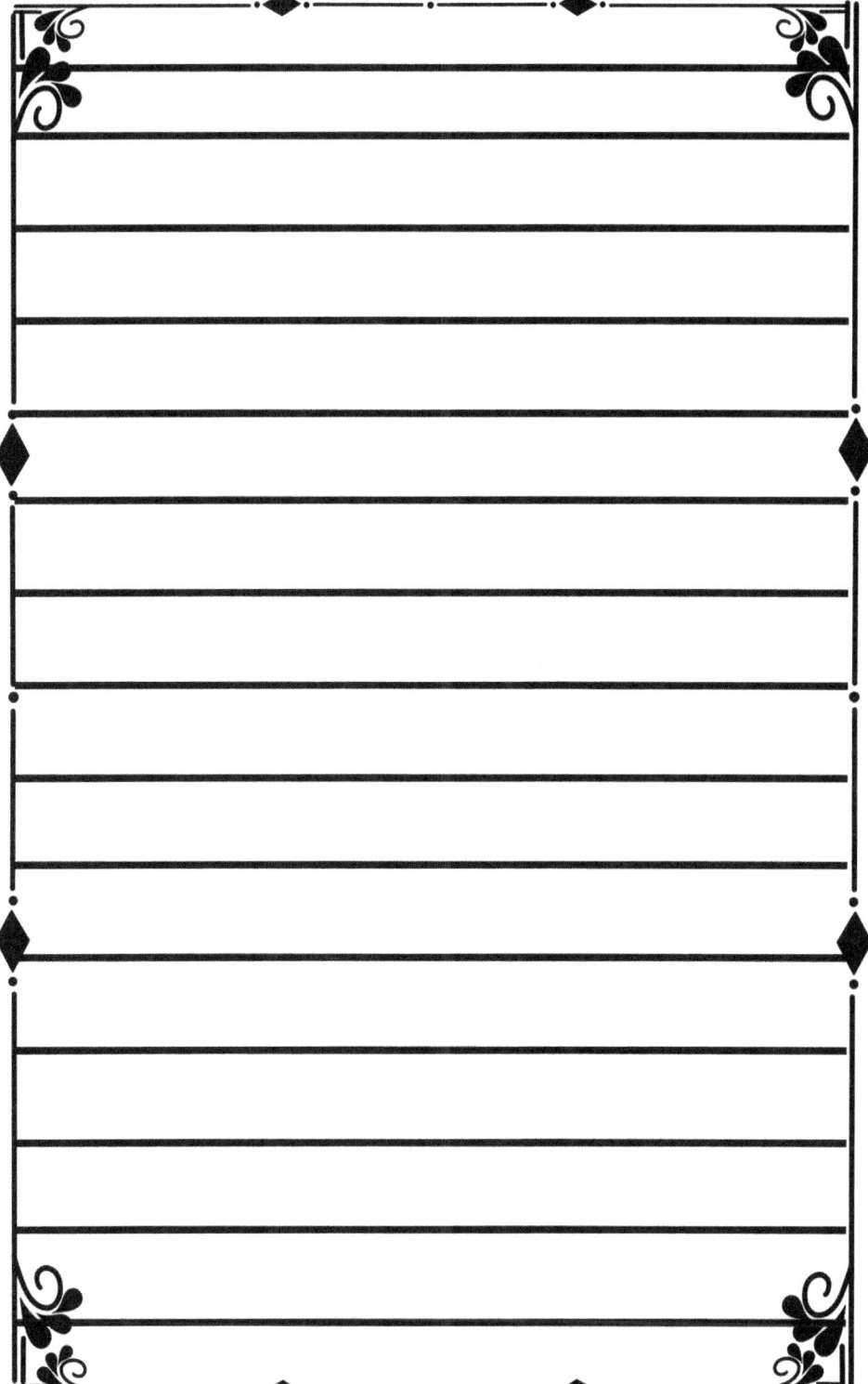

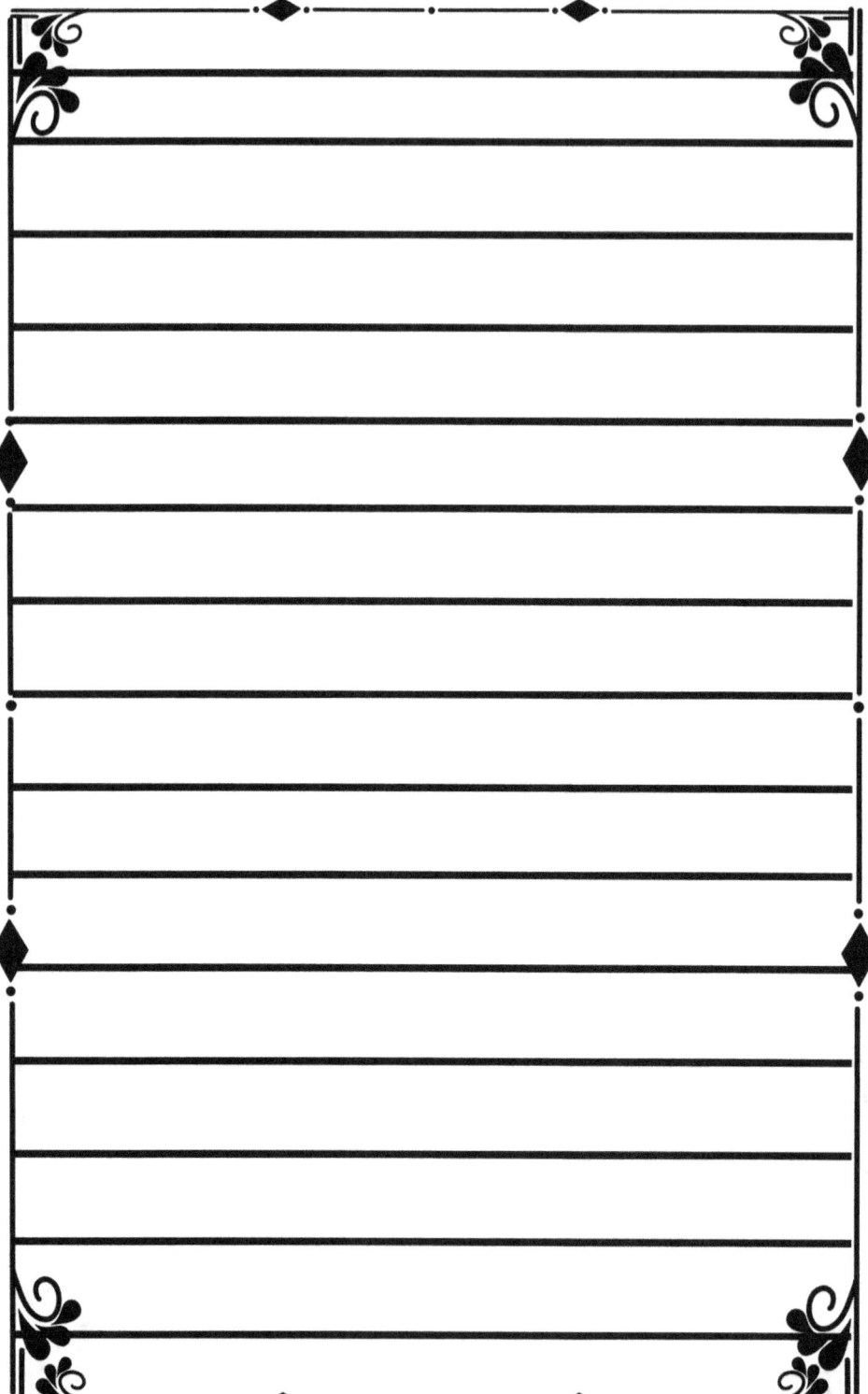

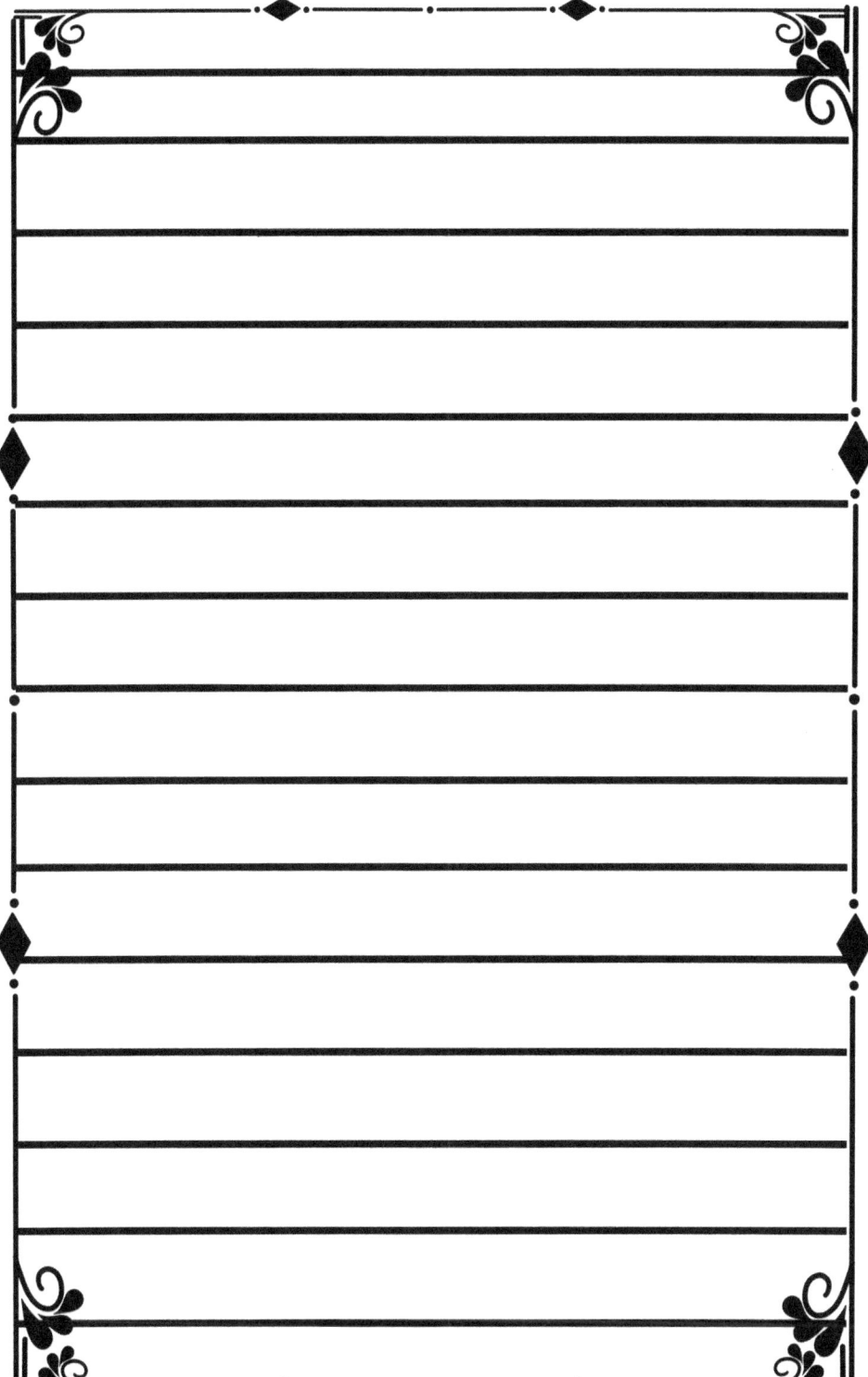

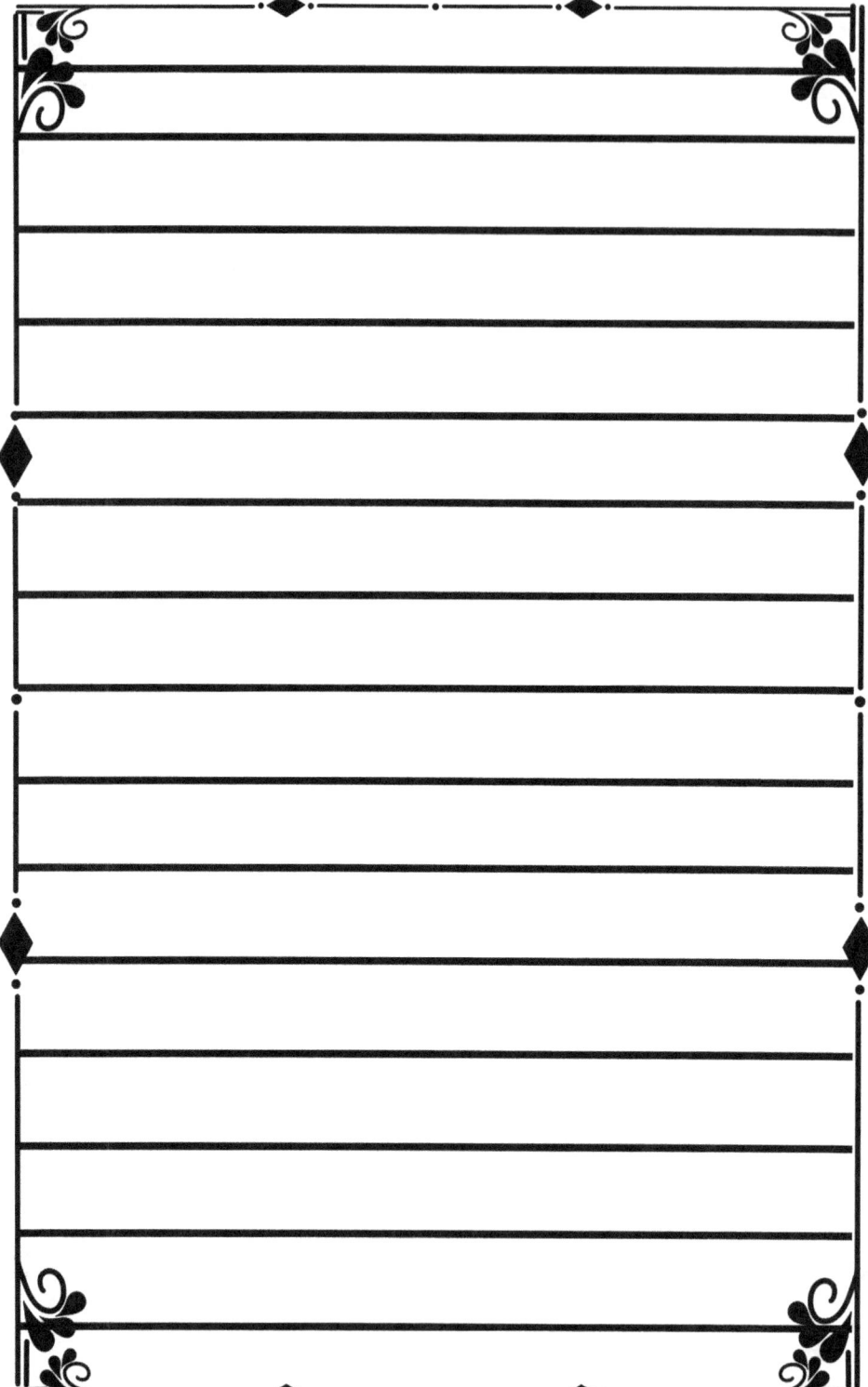

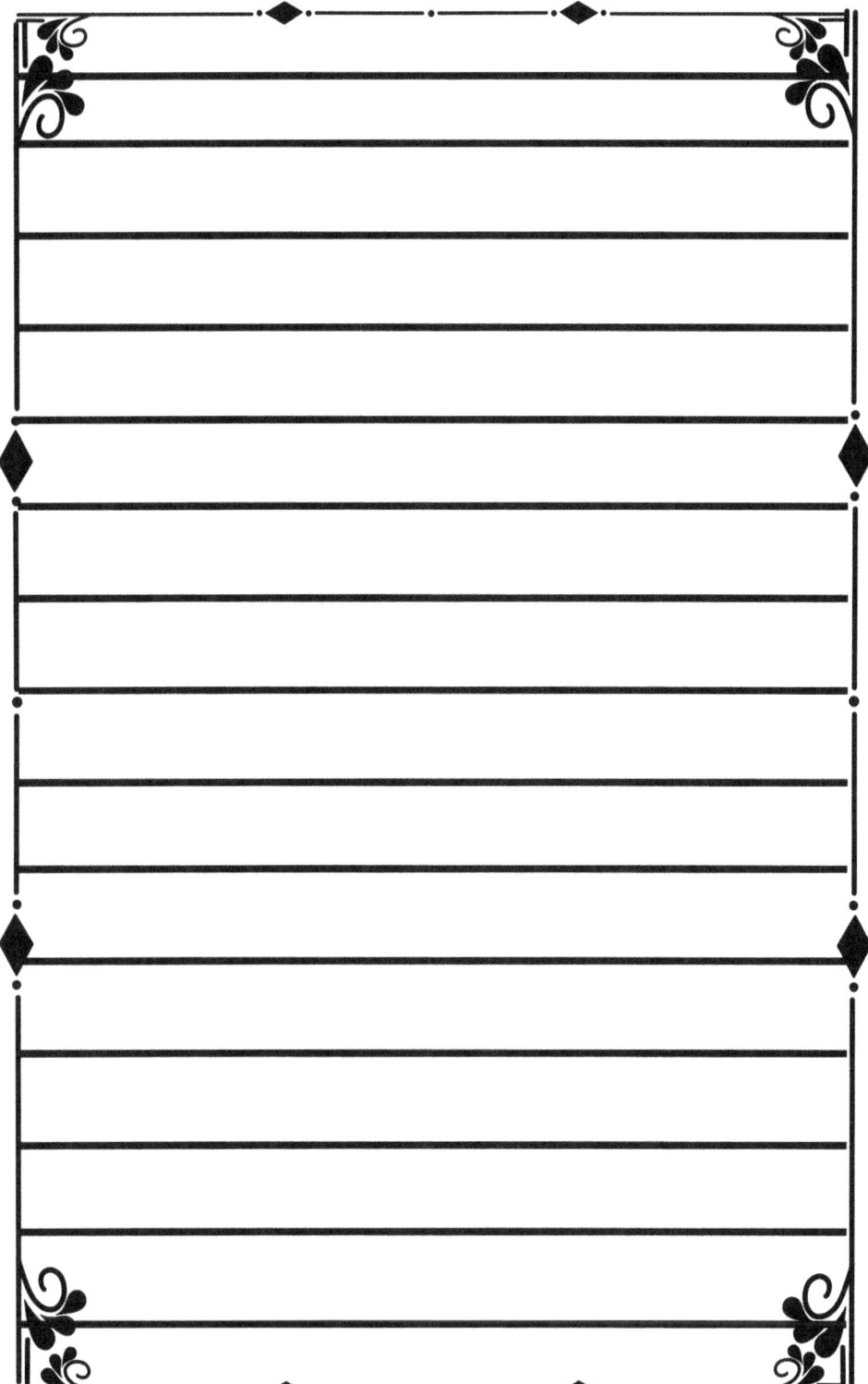

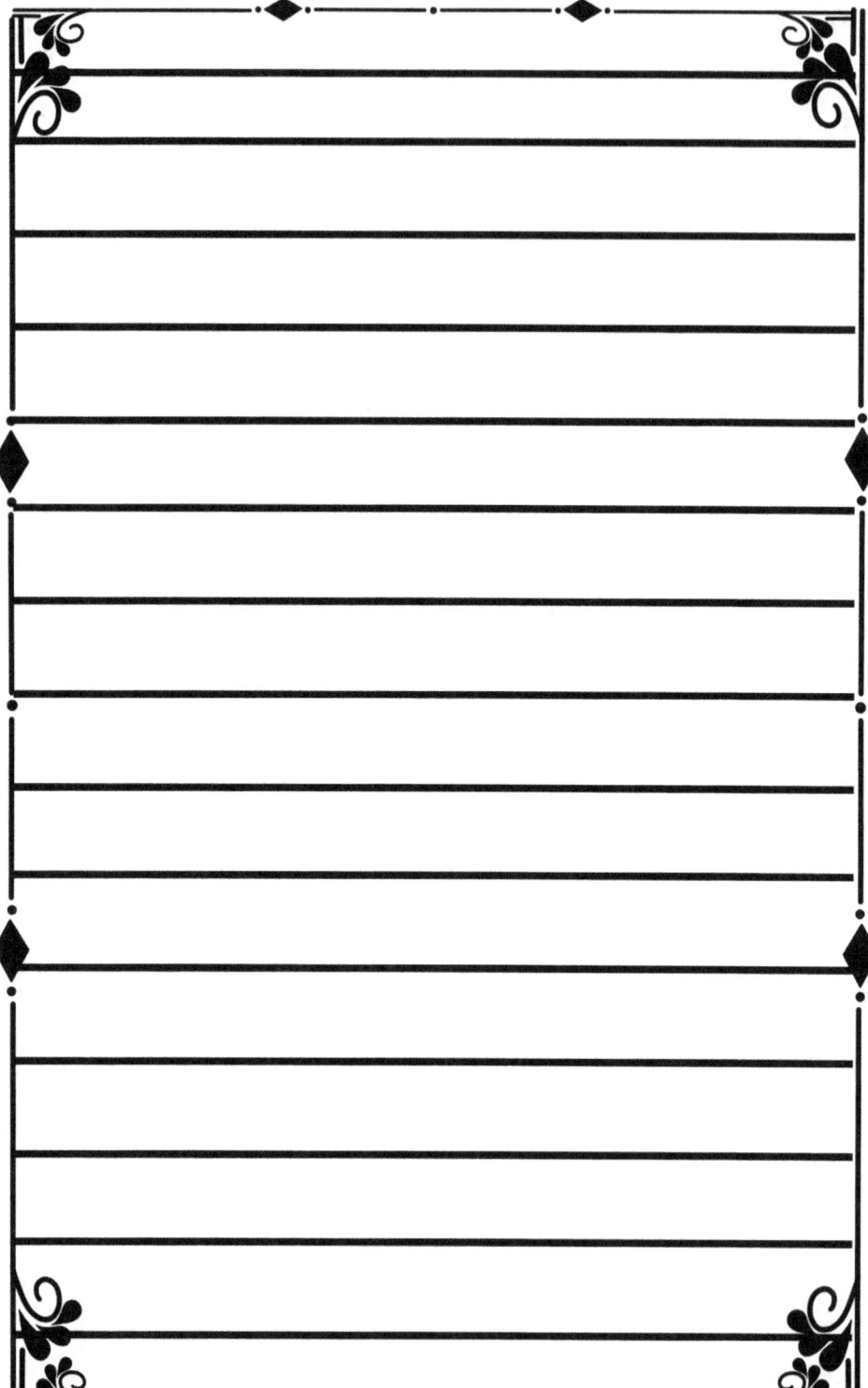

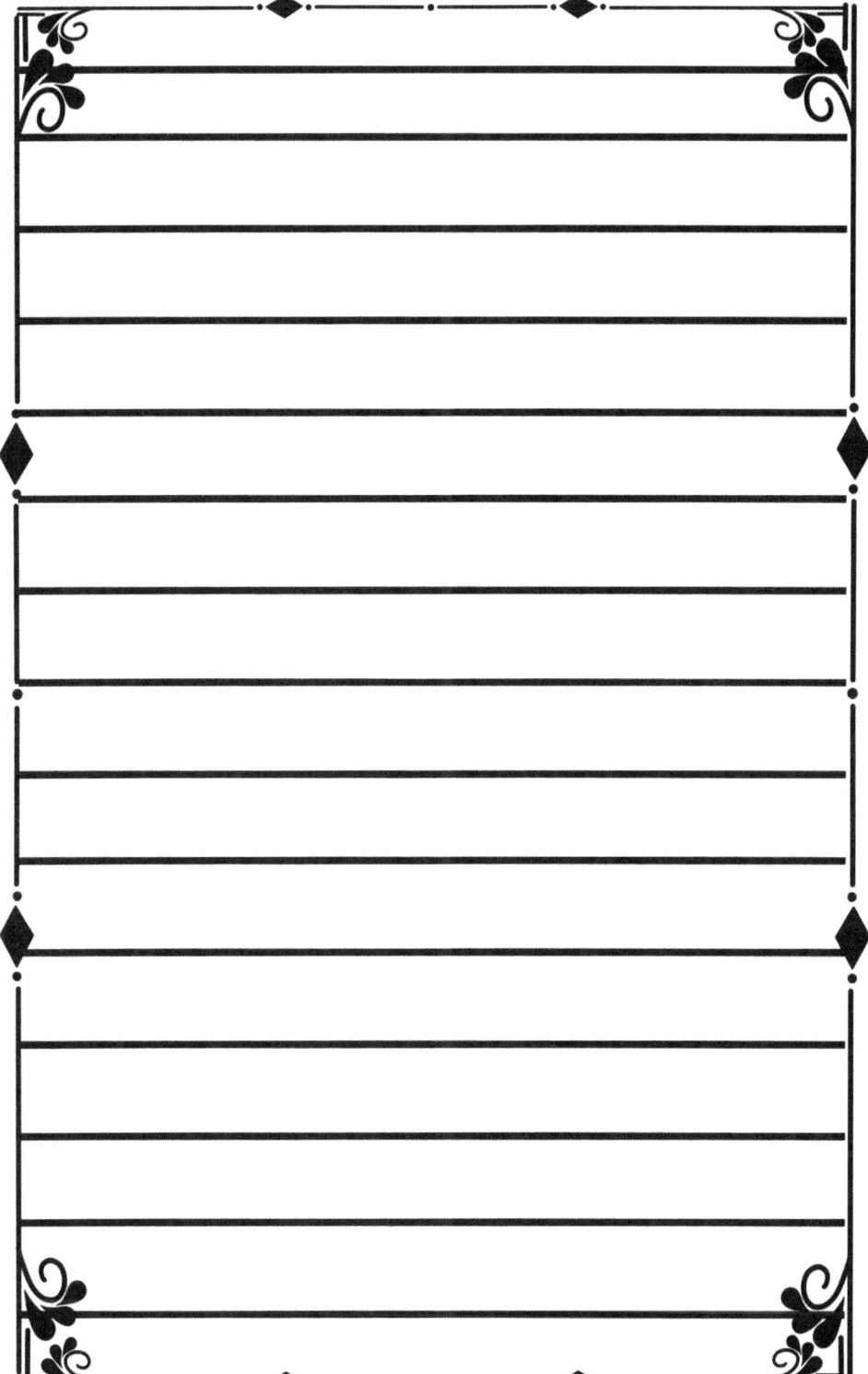

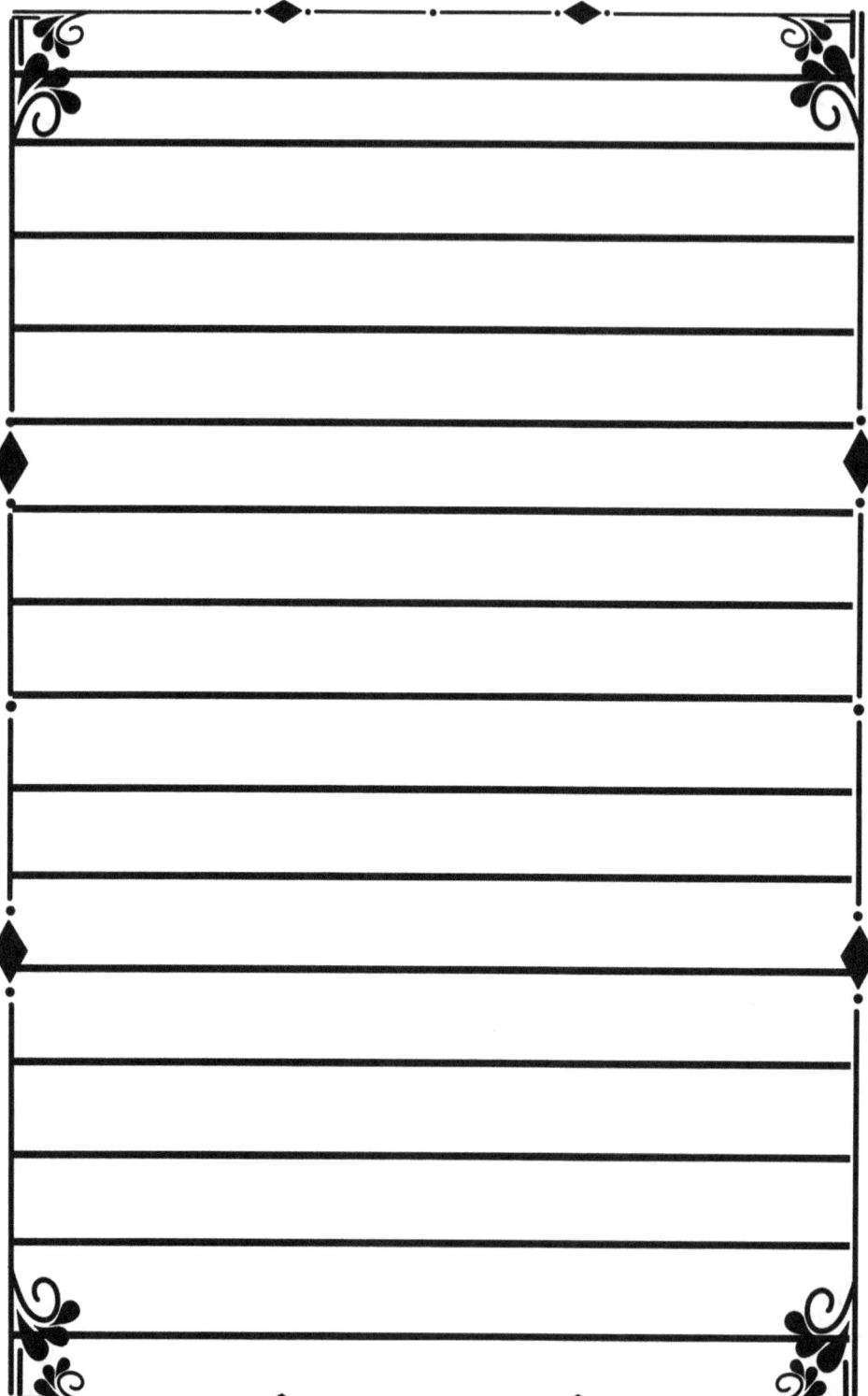

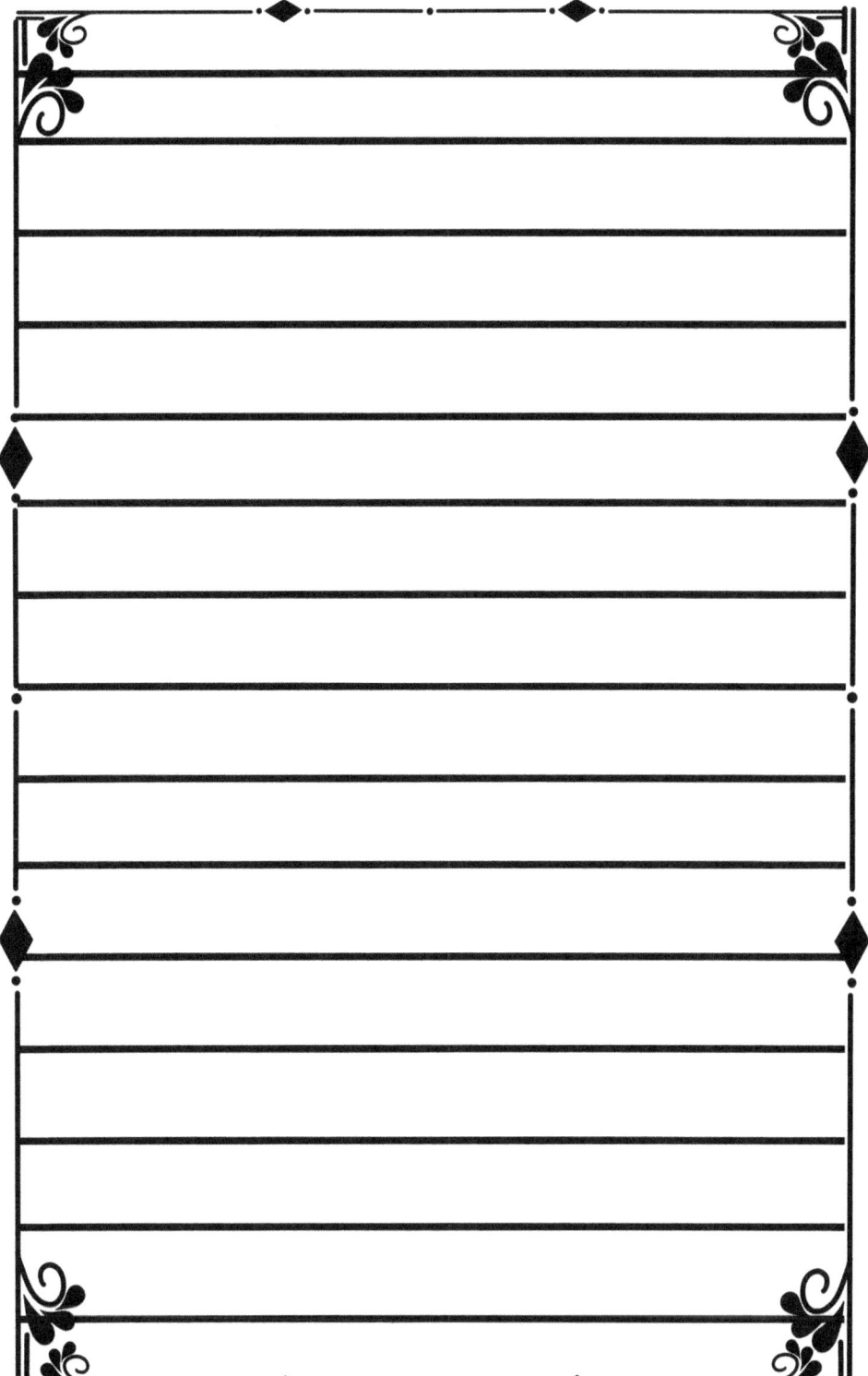

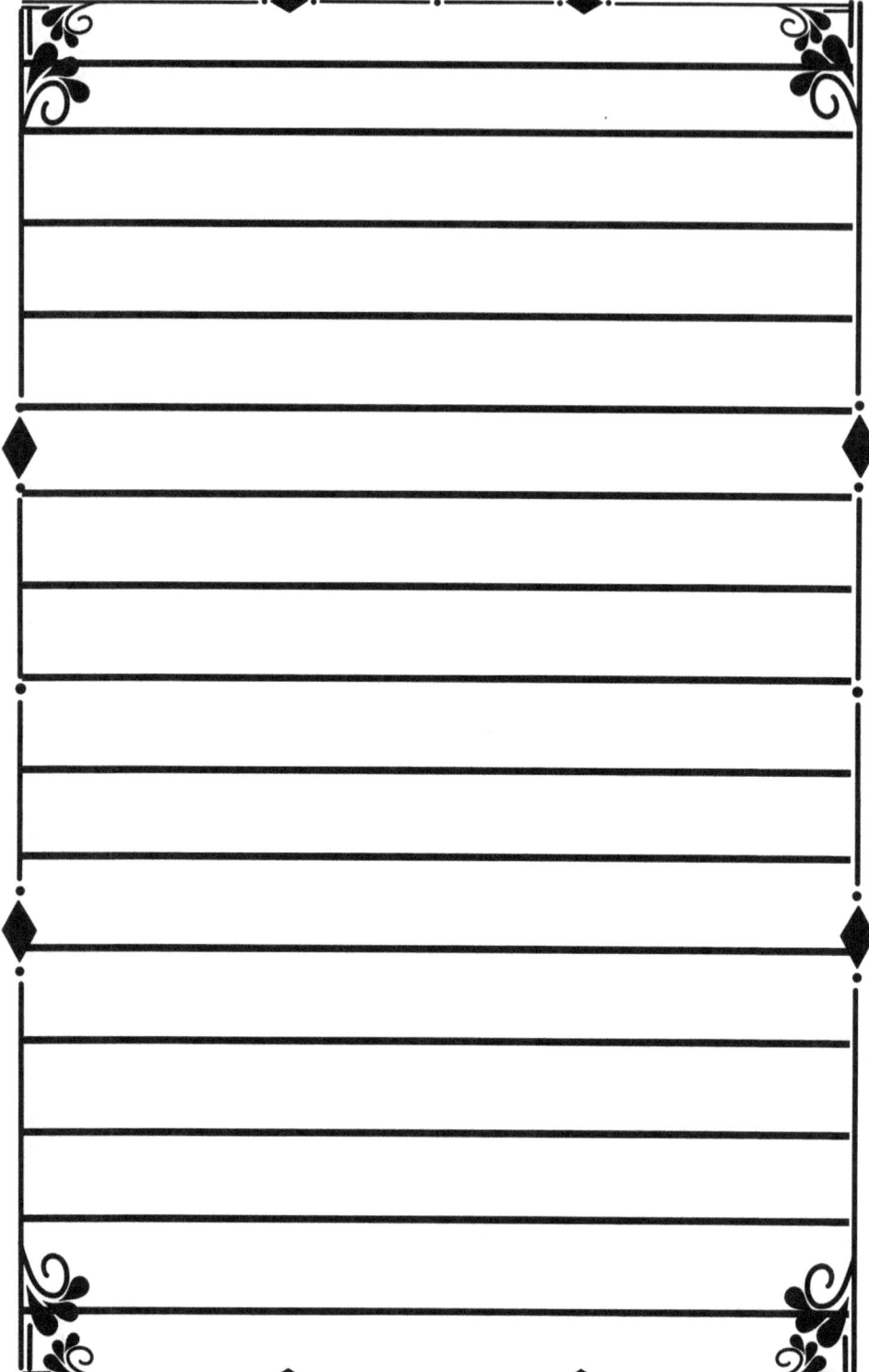

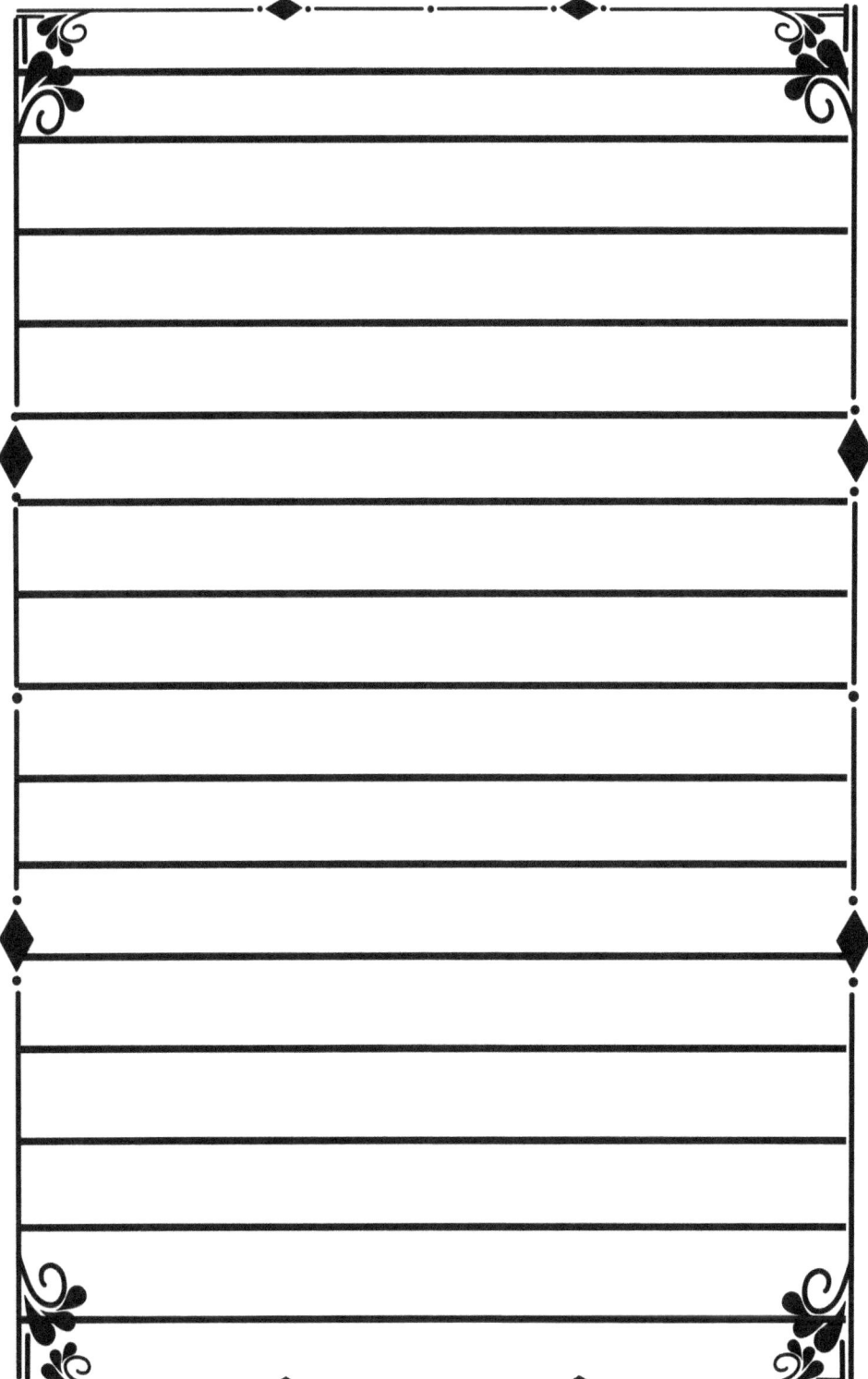

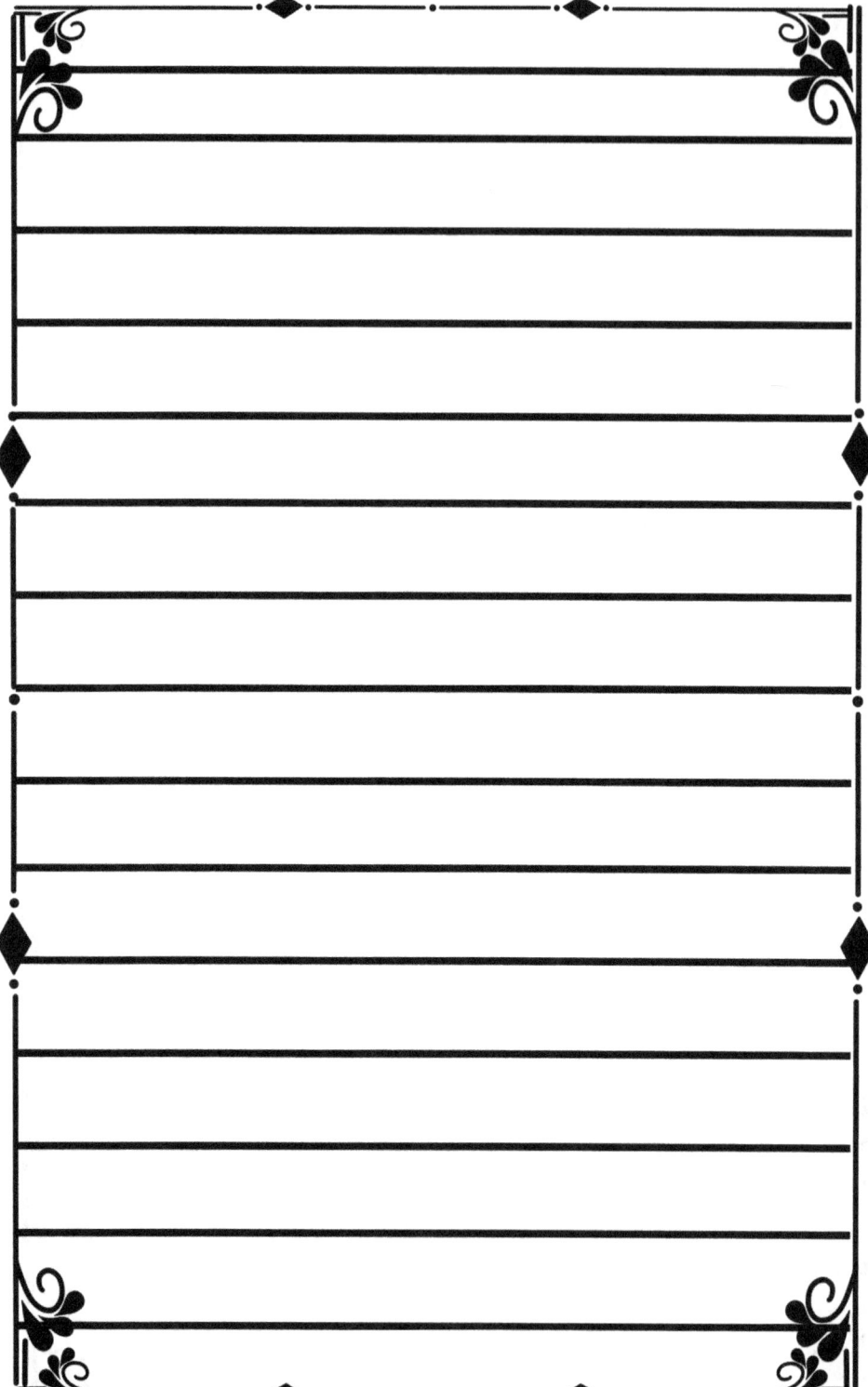

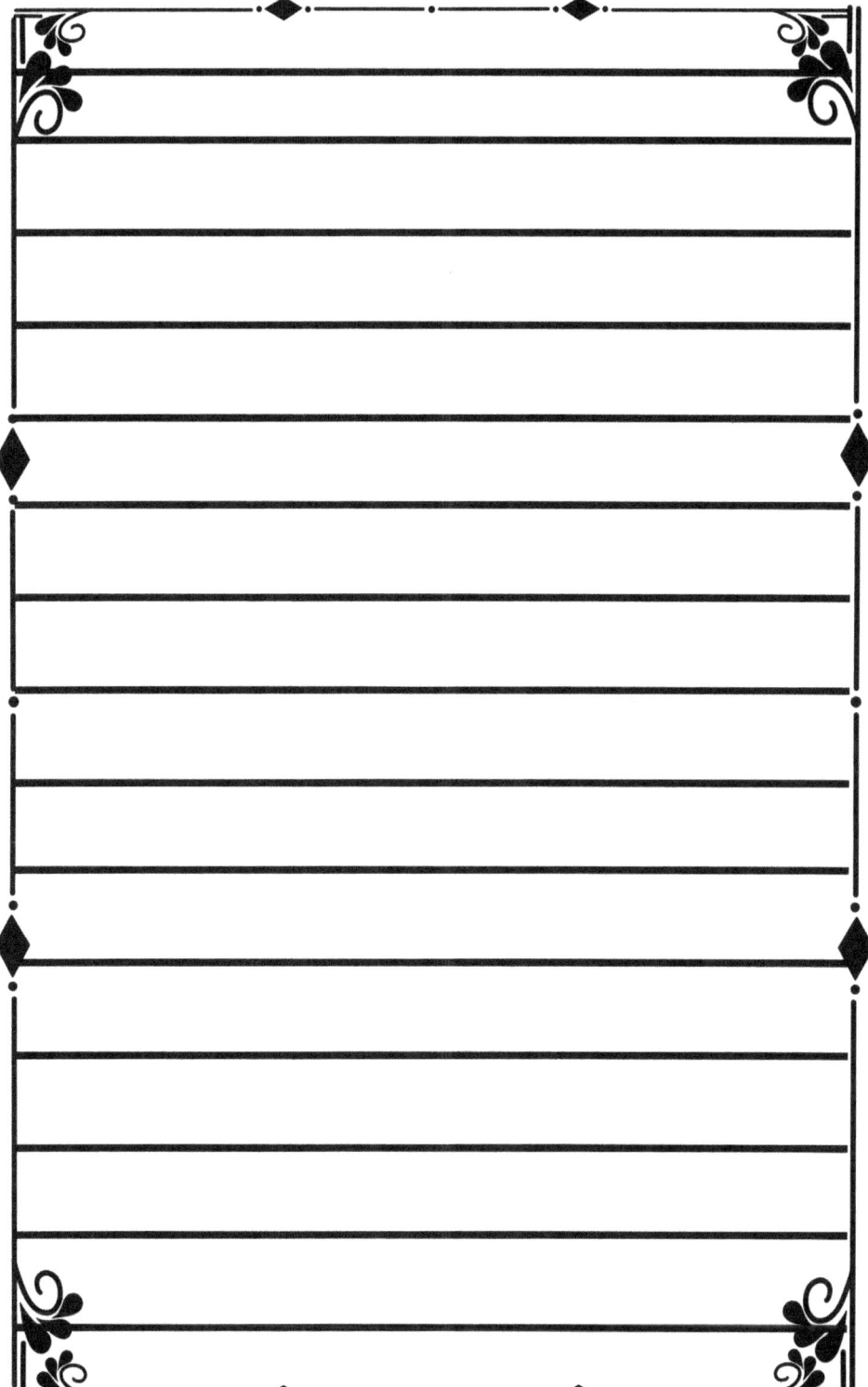

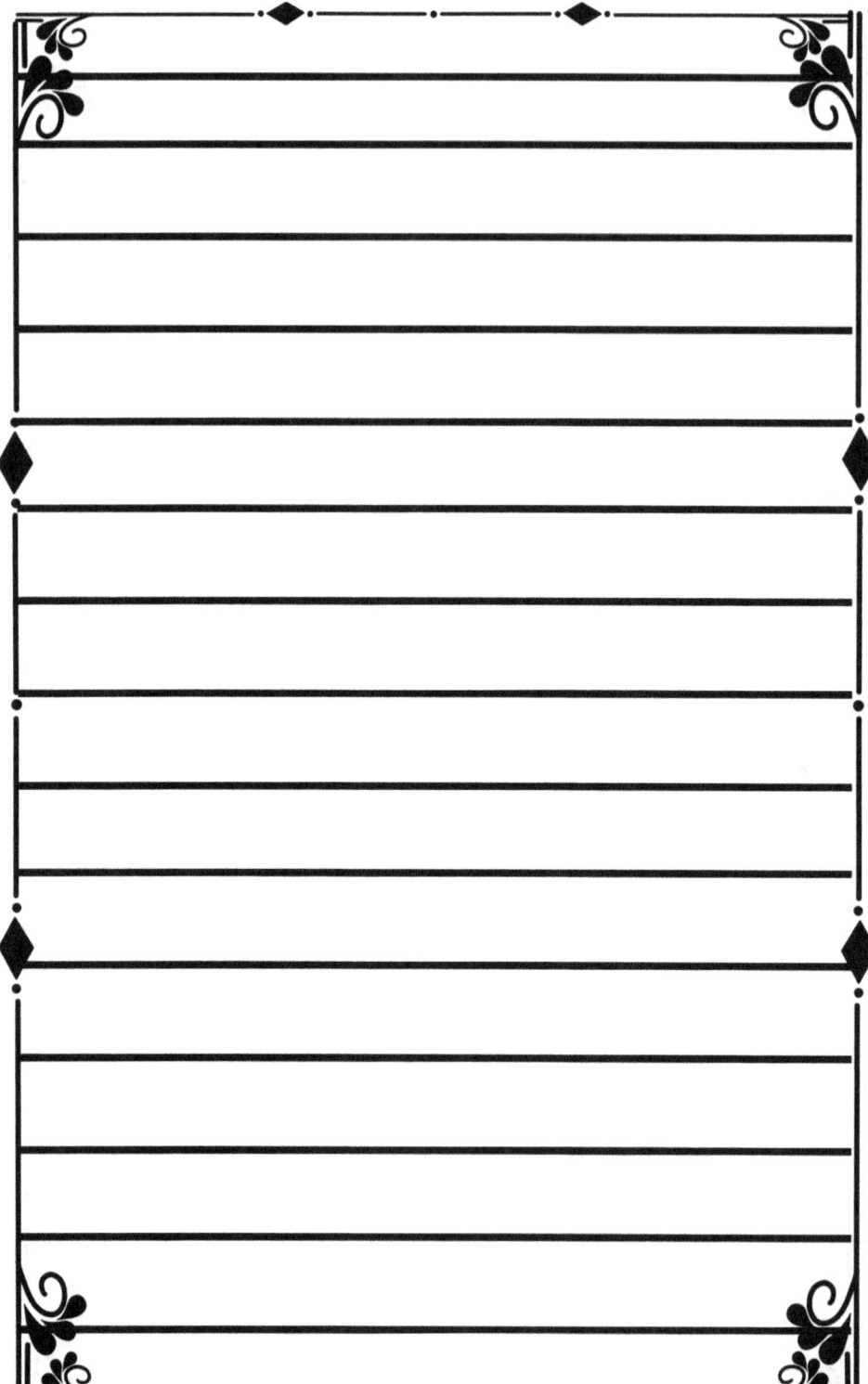

IN GRIEF, LOVE, CELEBRATION AND GRATITUDE

Today we are holding so much.

Today is my youngest brother's birthday.

It is Saturday. We slept in which was much needed.

We made time for the cemetery today. To see my dad. I really needed time there, in my thoughts and prayers. just there.

We cleaned the space a bit. and took in how different it is each time we visit.

Then we took a trip to see my mother-in-law, in the hospice care facility.

We spent two hours visiting her, and even our dog Griffin joined this time.

Today has been filled with soul care.

I wish to speak nothing into existence but I can't help but think and feel every time.... what if it's the last...

It remains true that grief, gratitude, and celebration all exist at once.

October 22, 22

How can you give your soul some care today?

IF MY MEMORIES OF YOU WERE A SLIDESHOW, WHAT WOULD THEY SHOW?

HOW HAS DEATH EFFECTED THE WAYS IN WHICH YOU TREAT THOSE WHO ARE STILL ALIVE?

HAS IT CHANGED YOU?

IN WHAT WAYS HAS THE DEATH OF SOMEONE, MADE YOU VIEW LIFE DIFFERENTLY? DO YOU LIVE LIFE DIFFERENTLY THAN BEFORE?

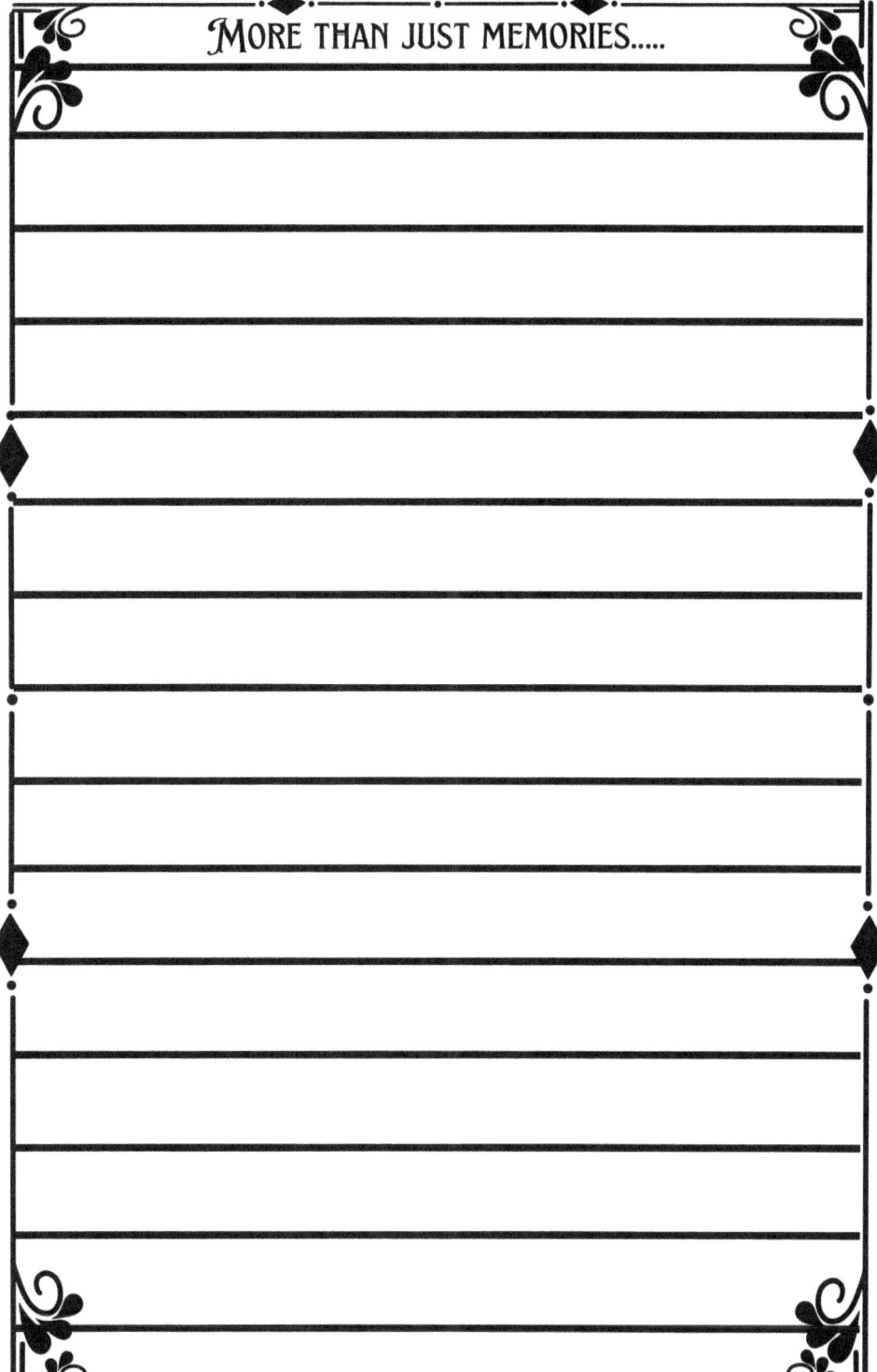

MORE THAN JUST MEMORIES.....

WHAT IS GRIEF?

Whew, that's a loaded question.

I think it's a mix of emotions and can be a variety of situations and show up differently for yourself and for others.

Grief and gratitude are very connected for me.

I feel that grief is a very human experience and it's a part of life.

It's a part of healing.

I think of balance and a caterpillar becoming a butterfly.

As a writer, I love feeling and experiencing and expressing.

I don't love pain.

But I do see everything as a learning experience.

Maybe we go through things to help others in some way
maybe we go through it for ourselves

Expression to me is writing, projecting my feelings, creating, the way I parent, speaking in community and listening.

I feel like the relationship between expression and grief can vary depending on who and what. Different situations vary. For me, my common ground is trying to allow myself to be honest and allow the feelings to be what they are.

I keep thinking of a caterpillar and turning into a butterfly. The transformation and breakthrough.

How some parts in people's lives can look so beautiful to others but that not everyone sees what it feels and looks like to get to that outcome.

That pain and grief can come in all parts of transformation, even in the happy times.

I feel like grief is something you move through but don't get over. For me it seems to be true.
Knowing my grief, doesn't help me help others grieve. I know I can't fix anyone and I don't want to. I am not in a rush to save anyone from their grief, as much as it can hurt me to see others hurt. I believe in feeling your feelings. I can't base someone else off of my experiences.

I think grieving well is allowing yourself to feel. To have your moment.

But what if that means- that these horrible things on the news come from people grieving?

No excuse, but what if we had more support around grief and feeling/dealing with our feelings.

What about a kid throwing a tantrum? What if how we are responding is us responding to their grief? Could we teach and model differently? What are we teaching? What were we being taught to experience/limit/make sense of grief when we were younger?

I am grieving so much.

I am grieving those who passed, those who are alive that I do not know (family), not knowing my "roots", having to move in July, pre-pandemic life, the life I created during the pandemic that is now shifted and still changing, time lost with our oldest/time we weren't given, time lost due to drugs and alcohol, unaccomplished goals, childhood trauma, scared dreams....

When my grief speaks to me, it is telling me: "I am here, we are one. we are a team. I am not good or bad- I am what you make of me."

*******Thank you Melinda C. Thank you for today's time together. "Loss and grief workshop"
Thank you for the questions asked.
I love being able to reflect, especially to listen to others and time to speak. What a beautiful space to be in.********
Due to privacy, I am only sharing my reflections

April 15, 2022

GRIEF IS THE MEMORIES I
HAVE LEFT
IT'S THE GOOD, THE BAD,
EVERYTHING IN-BETWEEN- ALL
THE THINGS I CAN'T FORGET.
GRIEF IS MORE THAN JUST
MEMORIES
MEMORIES, ARE MORE THAN
JUST MEMORIES- THEY ARE
EVERYTHING.
THEY ARE ALL I HAVE LEFT.
ALL THAT'S LEFT OF YOU. OF
US.
-----1/20/23

WHAT IS GRIEF?

FINAL OUTFIT

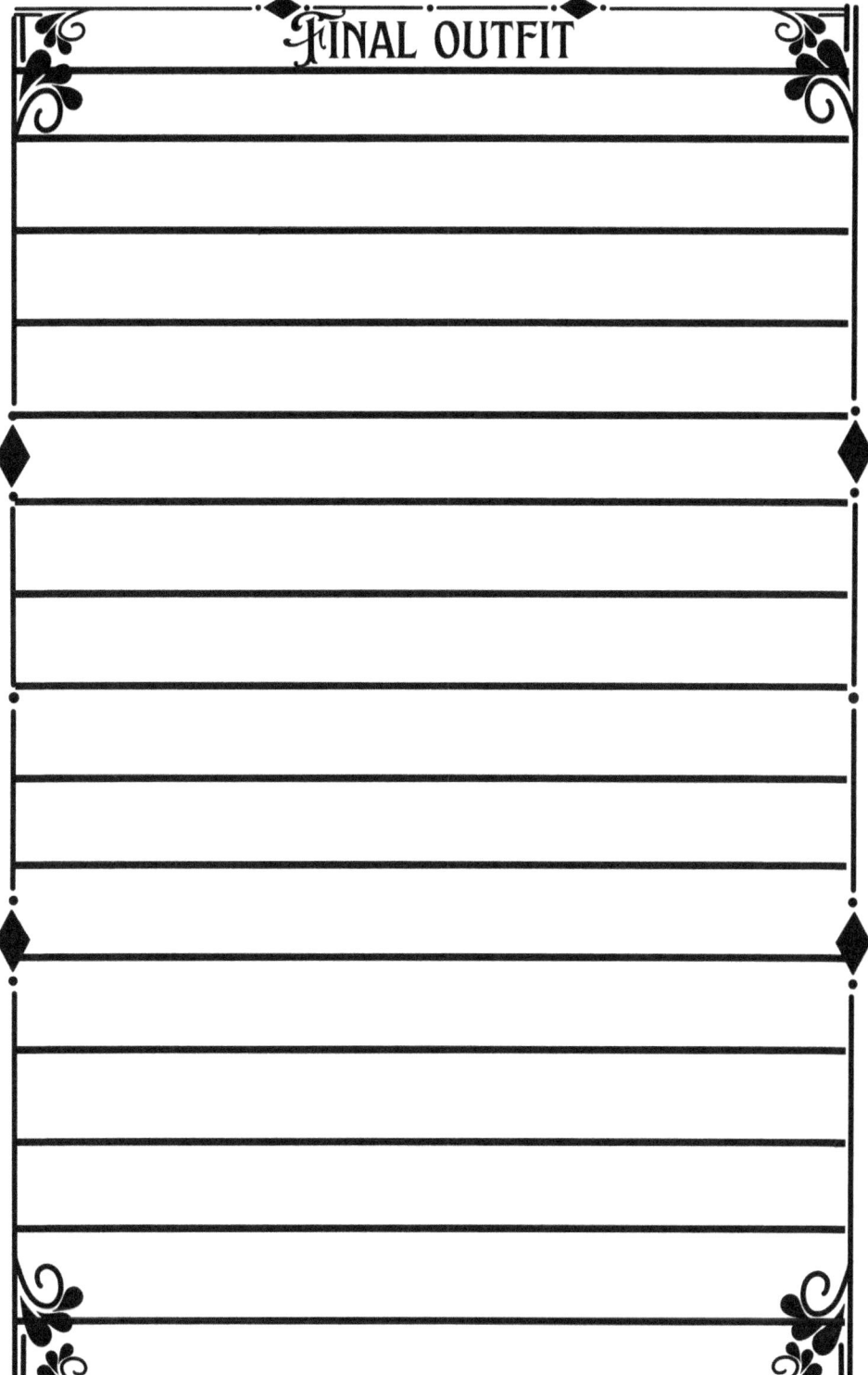

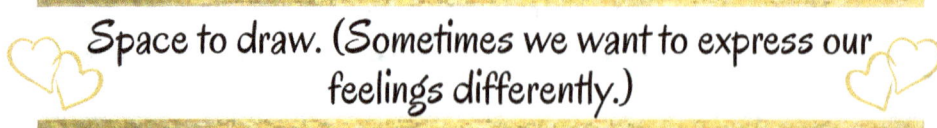

Space to draw. (Sometimes we want to express our feelings differently.)

HEALING WHILE HURTING

Thank you Susan M Lee Her.

I feel like I am always in need of healing and guidance.

For years I have struggled with supporting my ancestors with healing in the afterlife, supporting myself with the healing of their passing.

You said "don't fear what you learn today, embrace it"

"Today is your day. you are meant to be here"

The practice we did of closing our eyes and following your voice and words of actions to take. I can't even explain step by step.

I know that I could see everything so clearly.

Usually, I can't always see so clearly but more and more it's becoming different.

As we called in ancestors -names flooded to me: grandpa Robert, dad, cousin wayne, baby cousin, grandma madeleine, uncle john, Josie, aunt Denise, uncle larry.

I could hear and feel Jossie, my dad, and my uncle John. I could hear their voices and feel their hugs and see the light.

A single tear fell on my hand.

Then more.. it started getting hard to let go as if I was calling them back. I didn't want to let go. Even though at the moment I had.

....how do we create boundaries? was a great question

I thank you for the space you gave, for the energy, for that moment to happen. For your gifts and healing and your presence.

I felt like I wouldn't be ready for the next speaker.

I couldn't stop the tears and ground myself.

It took time.

Thank you for teaching us that anyone who passes is an ancestor.

Thank you so very much.

#popuphealingcenter day 4 on thankful Tuesday.

or should I say transformational Tuesday?

wow

—June 9, 2020

THIS NEW JOURNEY OF MINE, THAT IS NOT JUST MINE.......

THIS NEW PART OF LIFE, THAT IS THE END OF ONE'S LIFE.....

EXPECTED EXPECTATIONS

*We give ourselves expectations we expect others to
have of us
We think we know and we take actions based on a
thought.*

*"I can't take time off work"
"They won't understand "
But come to find out, they care more
They are human too and understand.
I am no good at work if I am a mess
I am better at work, after taking time to deal with
this.
Not only did my boss understand, but drove me to
where I needed to be
I didn't know about bereavement time, I wasn't
ready for this kind of grief.*

*"I just need a day" I remember thinking
I'll be back to work tomorrow.... What was I
thinking?
He never got better, everything happened so fast
I needed way more time- now I was cashing in on
sick and vacation.*

"I can't have a break to break
Because I need to be a mom, a wife"
I need to live life
Do you know what that's like?
To have all these "shoulds" playing in your mind
And yet it doesn't matter at the same time.

when life is taken
And your life is now different
And you no longer feel whole
Because now you are broken.

You have to move different.
I don't drink or smoke so that outlet is not for me
If I chose that now, it might be the end of my
story.

I need to write, document.
Feel it and be real
I need space, I need time, I need reflection and
help.

I have to take each day and moment as they come
That's the only way for this process to be done.
This journey is never ending
I will be forever be coping.

People who don't understand, can't
There's no fix-it for grief
There's no timeline for healing
There's no cure for this
Grief is grief.
You have to take it as it is
Make the best of it? Can't make sense of it

It's a big issue that people are expected to be
anything other than human
Trauma is trauma
Pain is real
Grief is a big deal.
Mental health matters
Let it all matter
Because it does.

It's ok to not be ok.

Some people don't know how to handle that.

Some people don't know how to respond to someone who isn't ok.

Not being ok isn't a crime, it isn't a disease or illness (I get it can have factors that do exist.)

But grief is grief

It can be heavy

Not being ok doesn't mean something is wrong with you.

Not ignoring your pain and choosing to feel your feelings- doesn't make you "different or difficult or weird or a problem."

And, in that same breath.... It's ok to be ok.

No one gets to tell you how sad you have to be, how fast you need to "get over" anything or when you should be healed.

No one gets to tell you how to feel.

I encourage you to allow help, seek help, find healthy ways to cope and to know you aren't alone.

12/7/21

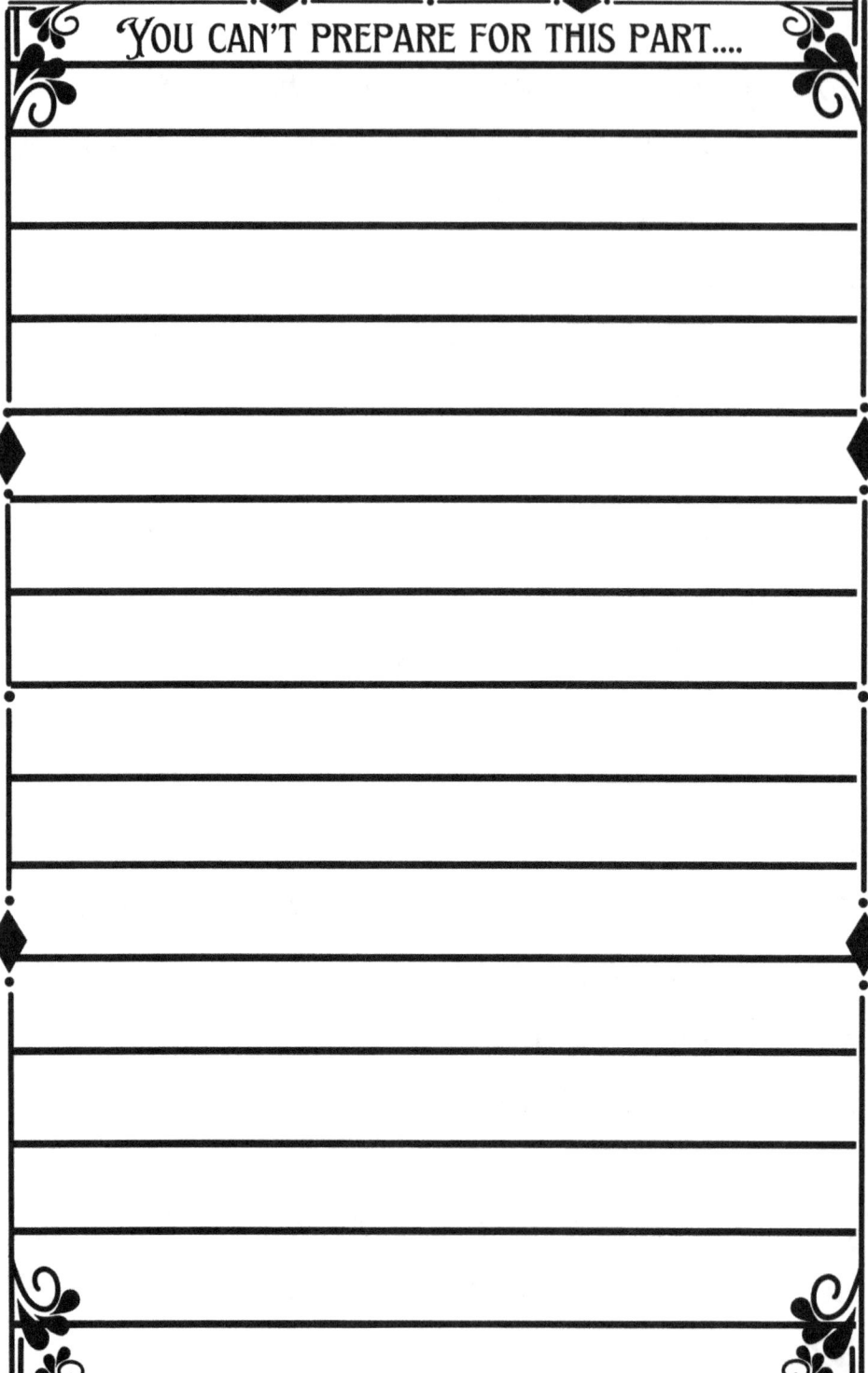

YOU CAN'T PREPARE FOR THIS PART....

WHEN WILL I BE NORMAL AGAIN?

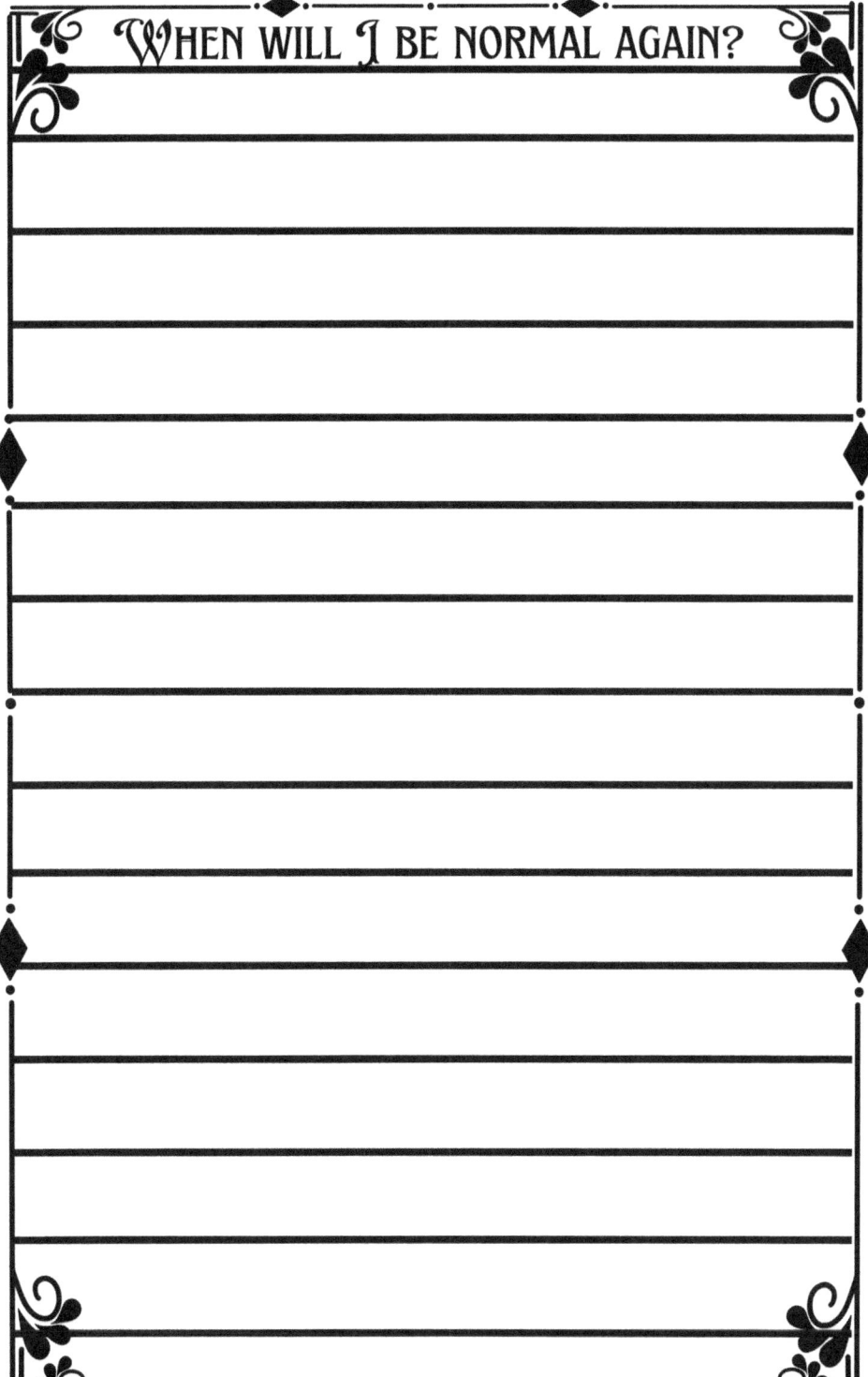

LEARNING TO LIVE AGAIN

MASTER OF GRIEF

I don't not feel like a master of grief.
I do not feel like I have closure or will ever.
The book I created was a big part of a peace I had never been able to reach before. It does not mean I don't still grieve or I am fully healed. It was definitely created from my pain and medicine for my healing journey.

I feel like right now, in this moment-in my life, the losses I am feeling are the losses of old stories. Old parts of me that I have outgrown or grown into. People and spaces that I have grown away from. Relationships due to the pandemic that have shifted or gone but I don't necessarily feel grief-because I embraced the good. The good of going inward and growing me.
The good from living dreams.

The good from growing from pain and making peace with surrender and change.

I don't feel like I ignore my grief or feelings. I feel like I feel my feelings well. That I allow myself to. Because I have been embracing the good, does not mean I have been ignoring the grief or hard stuff. I just created new relationships with me, my pain, my growth and my journey.

The pandemic has brought much grief. In many ways and layers.
Grief comes with not just death. But loss of relationships, self, jobs, homes, pets, things...ideas....
I am not all healed or fixed or done.
just because I am not feeling the way I used to.
February 23, 2022

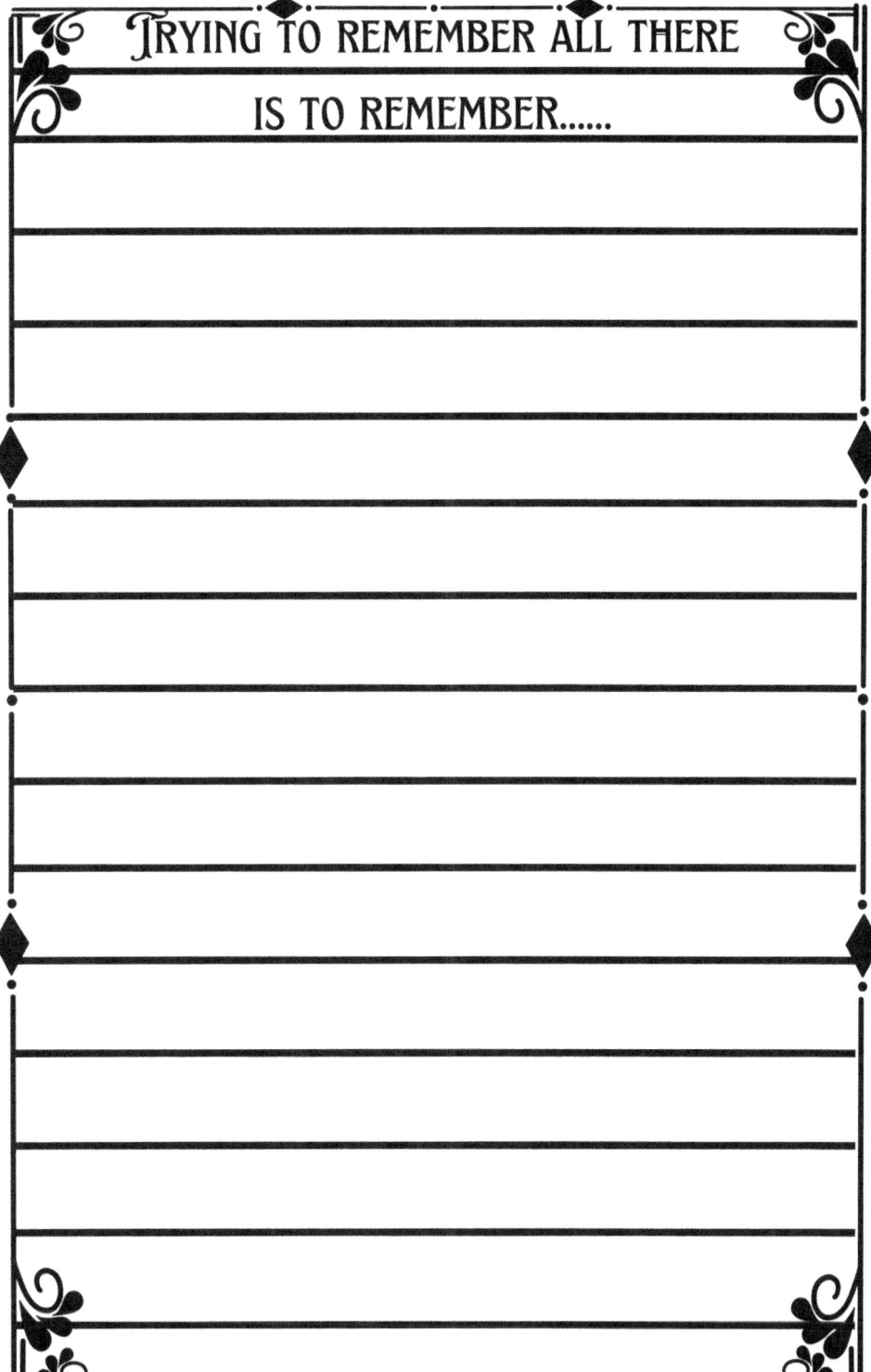

TRYING TO REMEMBER ALL THERE IS TO REMEMBER......

THE YOU, THAT YOU LEFT BEHIND......

Enjoying living this dream come true, book experience and all its journey that offers so much unexpected blessings

At the same time, it can be emotionally challenging re-living, re-visiting painful memories that are forever a part of me.
This grief and healing journey seems to be never-ending
But I am thankful for what it's given me
January 5, 2021

Today I have sat with all feelings:
Happiness, sadness, grief, anger, frustration, anxious, excitement, tiredness, physical pain, scared, hungry, full,
but of it all—gratitude

I am so thankful for it all. I am thankful to be able to feel, to deal and to know I am human.
I am not perfect. I feel shame, guilt-so many emotions.
March 15, 2021

(11/21/22)

When I made it home Friday from my afternoon shift, I was in horrible back pain. It's Monday now and it still hurts.

Immediately I thought "GOD wants me to rest" and also, I thought "of course, it would happen now- before the break- when I want to do so much. Just my luck. Is this karma?" I feel like it's another sign pointing me to the callings of my heart that I have been distracted from.

Thankful I am not working, because of such pain and wanting to heal and not get worse. Thankful for that.

At the same time, I am not happy about it happening at all.

I know before this year ends, I need time to grieve.

Gratitude grounds me and I don't run from feeling my feelings- but I have been moving forward fast. Moving forward but not moving on. I have so much to still heal from, learn from, and feel before anything else.

I want to take this week to find joy, peace, answers, and healing.

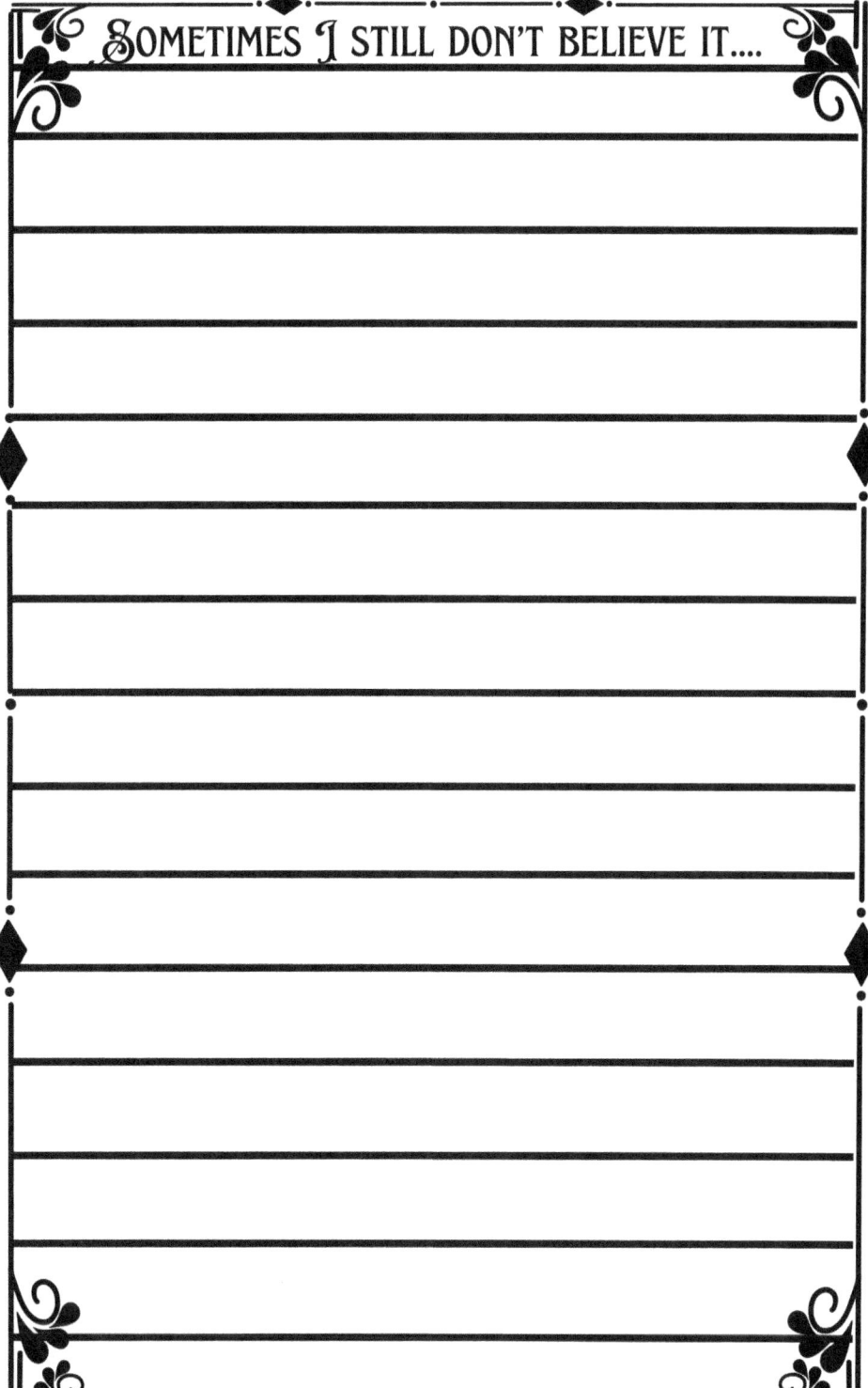

SOMETIMES I STILL DON'T BELIEVE IT....

Some space to draw or doodle. What does joy, peace and healing look like to you? How does it feel?

EVEN WITH YOU GONE, THE LOVE STILL GROWS....

I wish I could think of and be in celebration
mode, when I think of you
I wish it was that kind of mood.
because you deserve all the celebration and
praise
but grief just doesn't work that way.
because celebration isn't a celebration
without you here
and the thoughts of the future are empty
because the past is what brings you near.
all we have is memories
and some peace in the knowing you are no
longer suffering.
but that peace isn't fully peaceful
because heaven took a piece of my soul.

It is such a crazy reality to be living
to have so much gratitude at the same time
while grieving.

to have moments of laughter, followed by tears
to have anger, depression, strength and fears.
to have so many emotions happening at once
to have so many thoughts all wanting to be the one.
so much back and forth
so much pain, so much hurt.
so much disbelief
randomly the truth hits me.

sometimes the truth haunts me
sometimes the truth doesn't set you free.
or maybe that's ego talking
maybe I'm in denial about the whole thing.

the tears can begin to fall as quickly as they dry up
my voice can shake while the rest of me is held up.
sometimes my body can't stand, literally
sometimes the thoughts are too much for me.

to know you are no longer here
to know the end is near.
to not want to face the facts
to want your suffering to end while also wanting
you back.
cancer is the pandemic the world should stop for
I just feel like we need to do more.
cause more and more it's all around
you didn't deserve the journey of so many
rounds.
rounds of shots, medications and chemo
rounds of remission only to have it come back
and be told no cure would be so.

I wish I could celebrate you the way you deserve
I wish the grief didn't hurt.
but it does
and I have to let tears be enough.
it's all love,
it's all love.
September 30, 2022

THIS FEELING OF MISSING SOMEONE...FEELS LIKE...

TRIGGERED

Extra triggered, yelling more this week
on edge the past few days, tears flow easily.
trying to be patient with you
knowing I have to do my part too.

then today is here
the past days of chaos become more clear.

grief embedded in my soul
I don't need a calendar to let me know.
cause my heart is in pain
i go out with friends but it doesn't go away.

drinks, music, family
plans not going as planned but yet it's
flowing how it's supposed to be.
I allowed myself to be distracted
all to realize I can't be distracted.

the time always comes to face the truth
to know celebrations only include pictures
od you.

reminded that you are not here
reminded that time doesn't heal
wondering why am I here
wondering when I won't feel the way I feel
guilt, anger, pain and fear
release, gratitude, tears on tears.
9/4/22

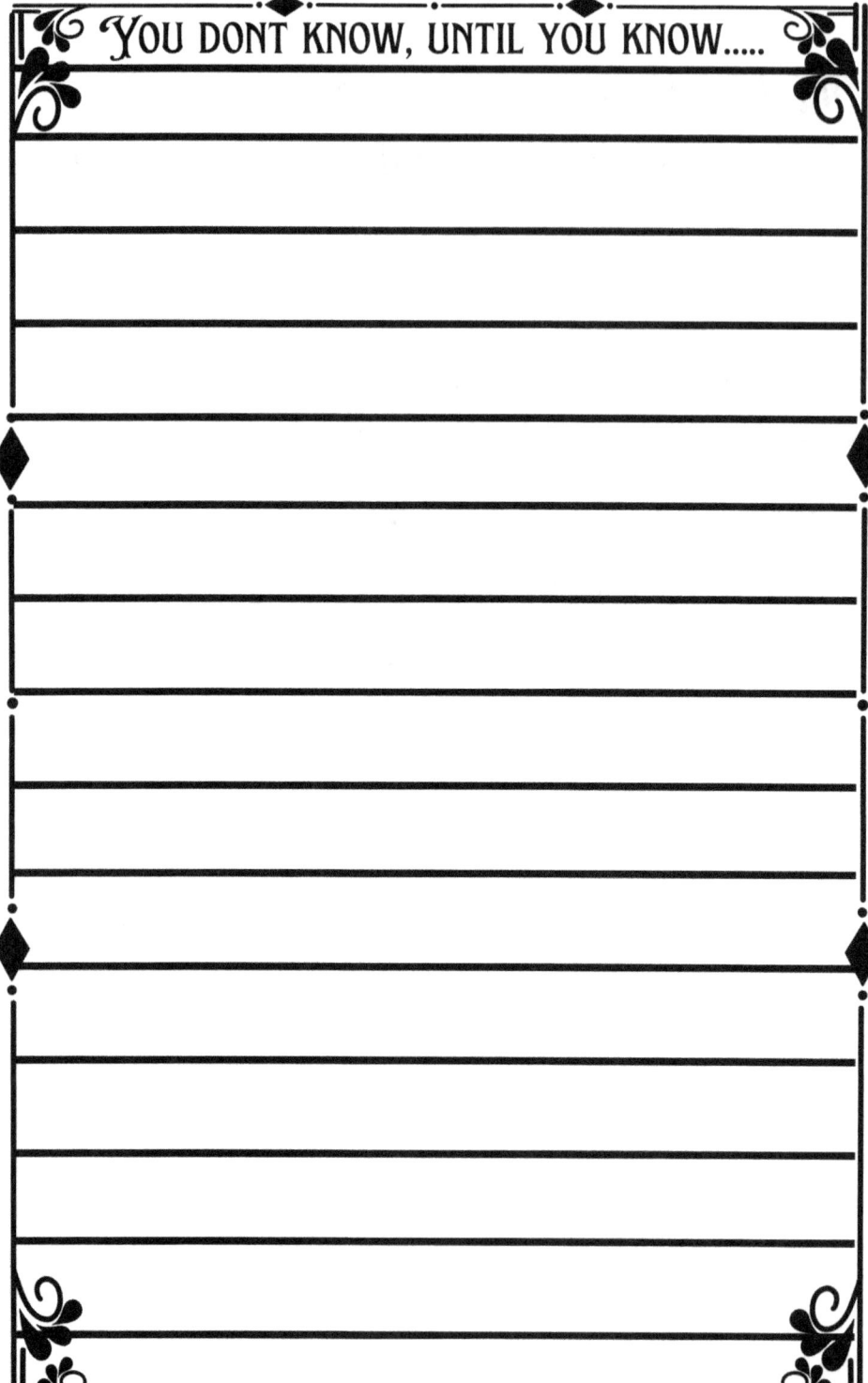

YOU DONT KNOW, UNTIL YOU KNOW.....

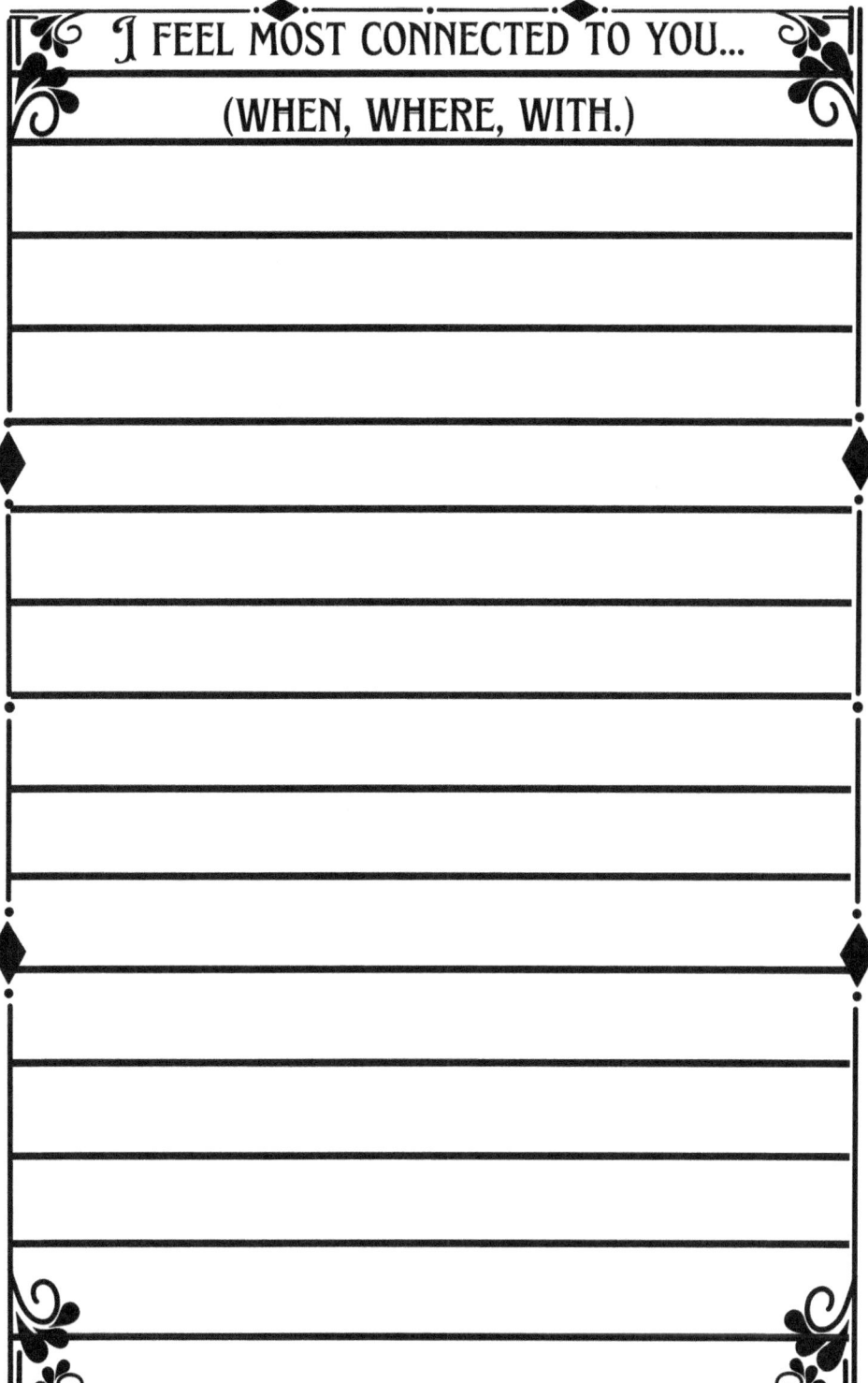

I FEEL MOST CONNECTED TO YOU...
(WHEN, WHERE, WITH.)

UNSURE

When my dad was taken off machines, I wasn't sure how long he would have. I prayed he'd make it on his own. I asked GOD if he didn't, then to let me know that's what was best for him- that he finds peace and choice and healing.

This wasn't during pandemic times, so we had a room full of people. Even a waiting room filled. I never felt so supported and yet so alone. I took comfort in knowing my dad was able to hear and feel all those around, that people got to say their goodbyes and pray together, that we were able to be a part of that transition and he wasn't "alone". There isn't any scenario that would make this easy.

I remember wanting to keep my dad warm. I was so upset we couldn't move to the comfort room; he couldn't eat or drink.

I wanted to rip those machines off of him so he could be peaceful

But I also knew those machines and things were keeping us together for this moment in time.

I remember holding his hand, saying I love him and I remember seeing when he left— it was how his face became peaceful (not what the machines told) and even then, I couldn't and didn't want to believe it. .....

I remember looking around waiting for someone to tell me he wasn't gone. That what just happened, didn't.

But it did. And I remember saying "NO!!!!" Really loudly. I remember saying to GOD that this isn't what I wanted even though I wanted him to stop suffering.

I remember not wanting to leave that room.

And yet leaving that room, I felt him leave with me. And I knew I had to get things done, quickly so he could Rest In Peace.

So I could find some peace....

Feeling these memories and emotions this morning

Praying for anyone struggling through grief and hard situations

December 19, 2021

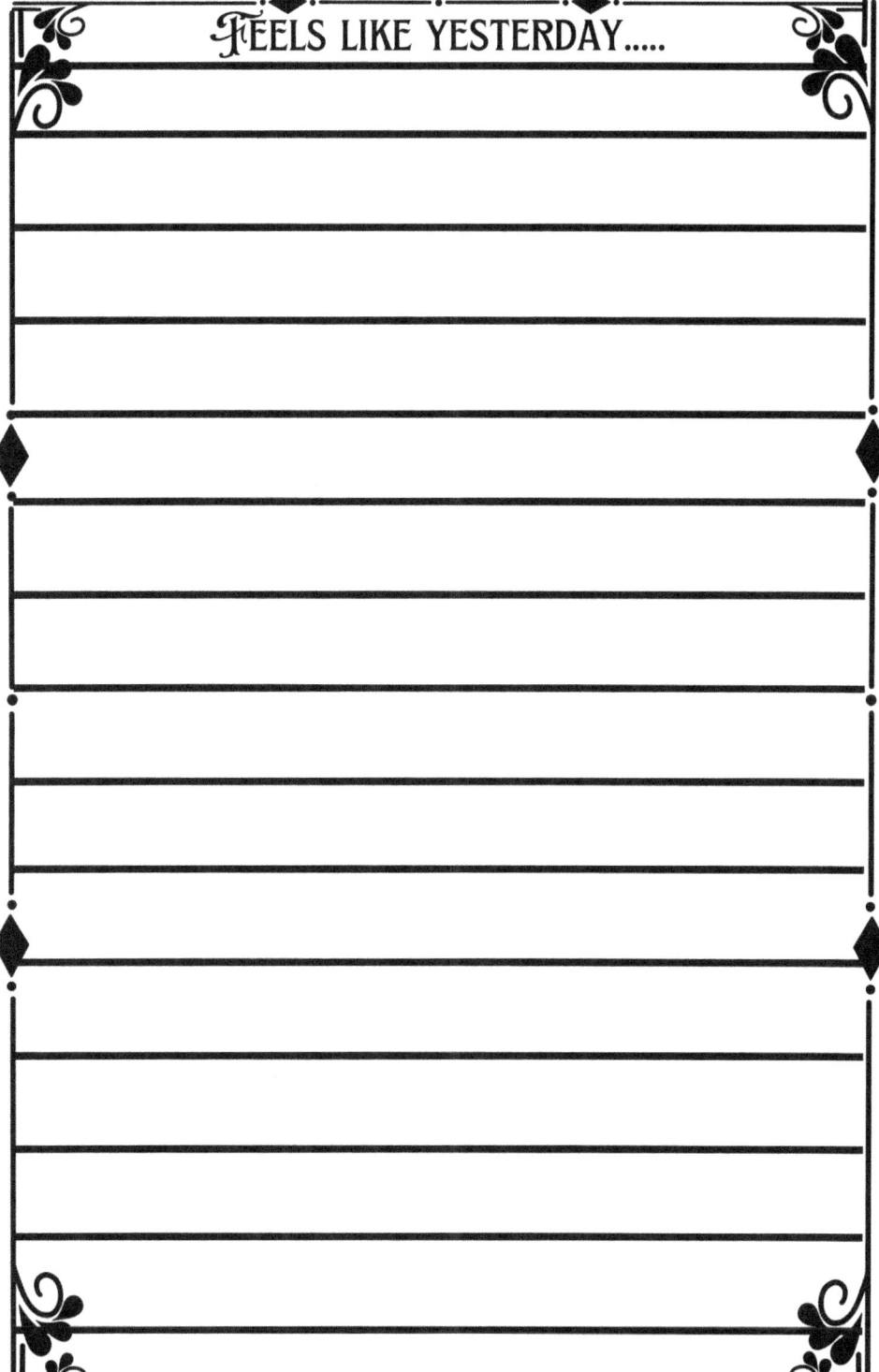

FEELS LIKE YESTERDAY.....

I spent the last 50 minutes with Robert S, whom I met during the "new year, love you summit.)

He is a cancer survivor and he is not only in the Doterra business but it is a part of his heling story and journey.

I connected with him over these two pieces, that have become such a big part of my life.

When I heard him speak during the summit, and he had a breakout room- it was the first time during the summit that I was not conflicted on which room I wanted to be in. I knew I wanted to be in his workshop, hearing his story.

It brought me to tears and lead me to his free gift of a zoom call today.

When I was in his workshop, I knew I was in the right place at the right time. That I was called and meant to be hearing him. I was reminded of why I should not give up on my Doterra learning and sharing.

I have lost my father and uncle john to cancer. My uncle and mother-in-law continue to fight.

I am not surprised to hear about healthy eating (organic), exercise, managing sleep and rest, finding the right doctor and support people- matter.

Essential oils, detoxifying, intermediate fasting- are extra steps that work for so many.

I wish I was on this healthy journey long before my father passed. It's been 8 years today and all I felt then was that chemo and things weren't for him. That I wished we found more natural ways. I wish I was able to give him a piece of my liver. I knew then that I believed in more than what were told to trust and believe. The fact that he had so many medications to take, never sat well with me. But I am no doctor.

I believe all of these other pieces are essential for all. Cancer or not. Sickness or not. These past few years I have been so focused on my mental health, inner healings. Other approaches, prioritizing sleep, eating better (I'm not perfect.

It's come with changing my mindset and habits and lifestyle and relationship with money-so, I still have a ways to go but I am changing and embracing that.) Movement, more natural cleaning products and more- have all been on my mind and heart.

Ever since my mother-in-law got sick, I have felt all of this the same, and more. but again, that voice of "who am I?" I just encourage everyone to speak up, because I believe we know our own bodies and stories best. I have learned I am in control of no one else. We can live in our truths and paths and keep going.

I intentionally made my call with Robert, for today. On my dad's anniversary. Because I just knew, it would help me on a day that's always been hard for me. I didn't know how but I just felt called. And, I am so happy I did. Because on my healing journey, this connection feels right. I am so thankful to learn more, be further inspired and have more support.
—January 21, 2022

WHAT DO YOU FEEL CALLED TO?

BUCKET LIST.... (WHAT DO YOU WANT TO DO IN THIS LIFETIME?)

HONESTLY....

I started feeling it earlier this week, when I realized what this Sunday would be....

When I noticed the grief attached, I steered away from it. Decided not to feel into it or think about it, at least not until the day got closer.

well, so much has taken place this week to keep me distracted.

but, tomorrow is still tomorrow.

mothers day.

For me, as a mother of 4.

Mothers day feels like it will forever be incomplete.

It will never be what I wish it could be, look like or feel like.

Because, for one of our children—although I am mom....

I am "step-mom"

and reality for us is, mothers day is not mine or our day to be together.

when sharing a child, many and most holidays are shared or switched off yearly.

One family always "misses out".

I have gotten used to celebrating holidays on different days.
getting used to it, doesn't mean it doesn't hurt or doesn't get to me.
I have my moments.

no matter the bond, the time, the love- that I know is shared between us all.
even with knowing I'd never want to take away from any mother.
I still have a piece of me that wishes I could have some of the day.
I will forever cherish being able to wake up to all of my kids and my complete family. even if only for hours or minutes or moments.
I am thankful my husband and I have both of our mothers.
I will be thankful for all that I am thankful for.
But, I will also allow myself to be human.
and the human parts of me feels all of these things.

Tomorrow is just another day to me.
I remember telling myself to never get to that point,
of feeling like "just another day."
but, the day before the day has become "my day."
and today has not gone as planned, with covid and
what not.
but, such is life.

I am forever thankful to be a mom, their mom.
honestly, I always wanted to be a mom and knew I
would be.
from the moment I heard he was in the picture—
our first who wasn't and would never be
biologically mine. I chose to stay. I knew nothing
but love.
and the love has only grown.
even if the choice and love comes with all these
other feelings at times.

I love being a mom.
being their mom. ....and now, we have a pup who
gave us a scare recently and definitely feels like
another one of my children.
May 7, 2022

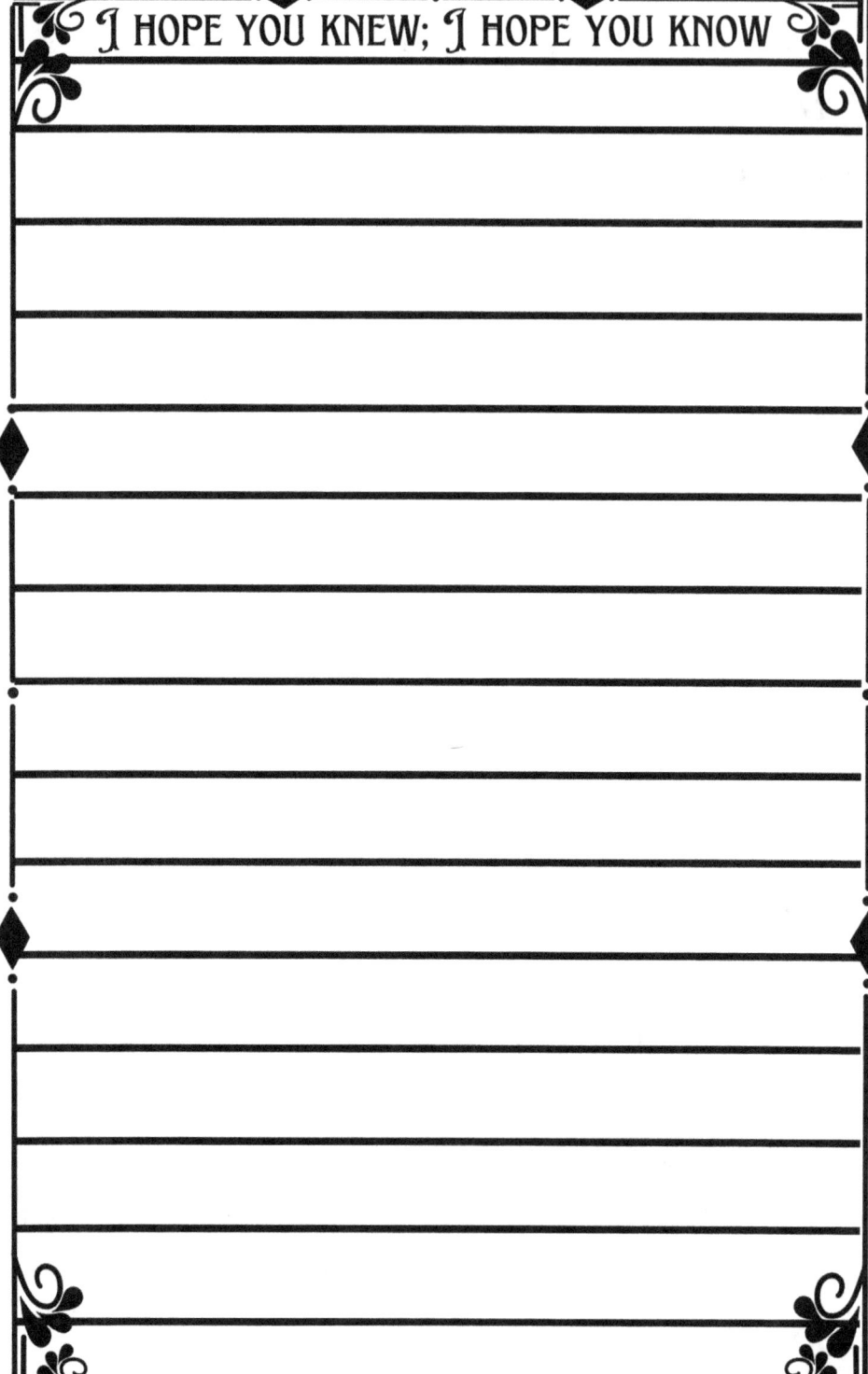

I HOPE YOU KNEW; I HOPE YOU KNOW

Touching lives, still

When my books first came a couple of days ago and my family was interested. I did think for a moment "I should be giving these for free, to all these people"

but if I did, I would not have made anything to buy more.

I am proud of me for "charging." Donation based, gifts, trades.

I am proud that my family has all paid, gladly.

I am even so thankful and proud that a couple have refused to not pay, even though I had a couple in mind that I was able to give to.

I love that people love me and are helping support this journey just because of their love for me.

I also love that those who are reading, are happy with their purchase for different reasons. I love that people are interested in what I created.

This morning my uncle told me how proud he is. And I felt like I could feel and hear my dad, but I just soaked in how proud my uncle is-he is very much a father figure in my life. I love that he brought up things I wrote about. I love that he read the book.

I love that he shared about his tears when reading. And shared how long ago the last time it's been since he's had tears like that. I loved all the honesty; it was all positive. I would have been happy even if it wasn't. I am just so thankful for the moment we got to have and the conversation. He brought up memories with my dad, and with uncle john and more. I loved it all.

I am so filled with gratitude, happiness and pride.

I am so filled with life. with hope. with wonder and just goodness.

My mom said she fell asleep reading again and that she only has 6 pages left. I can't wait to hear more from her. I am so happy that she is proud. I am so thankful that she is taking the time to read. She doesn't read books and yet she is reading mine.

What a beautiful last day of 2020. Just from these moments.

hey dad, you are touching lives. still.

——December 31, 2020

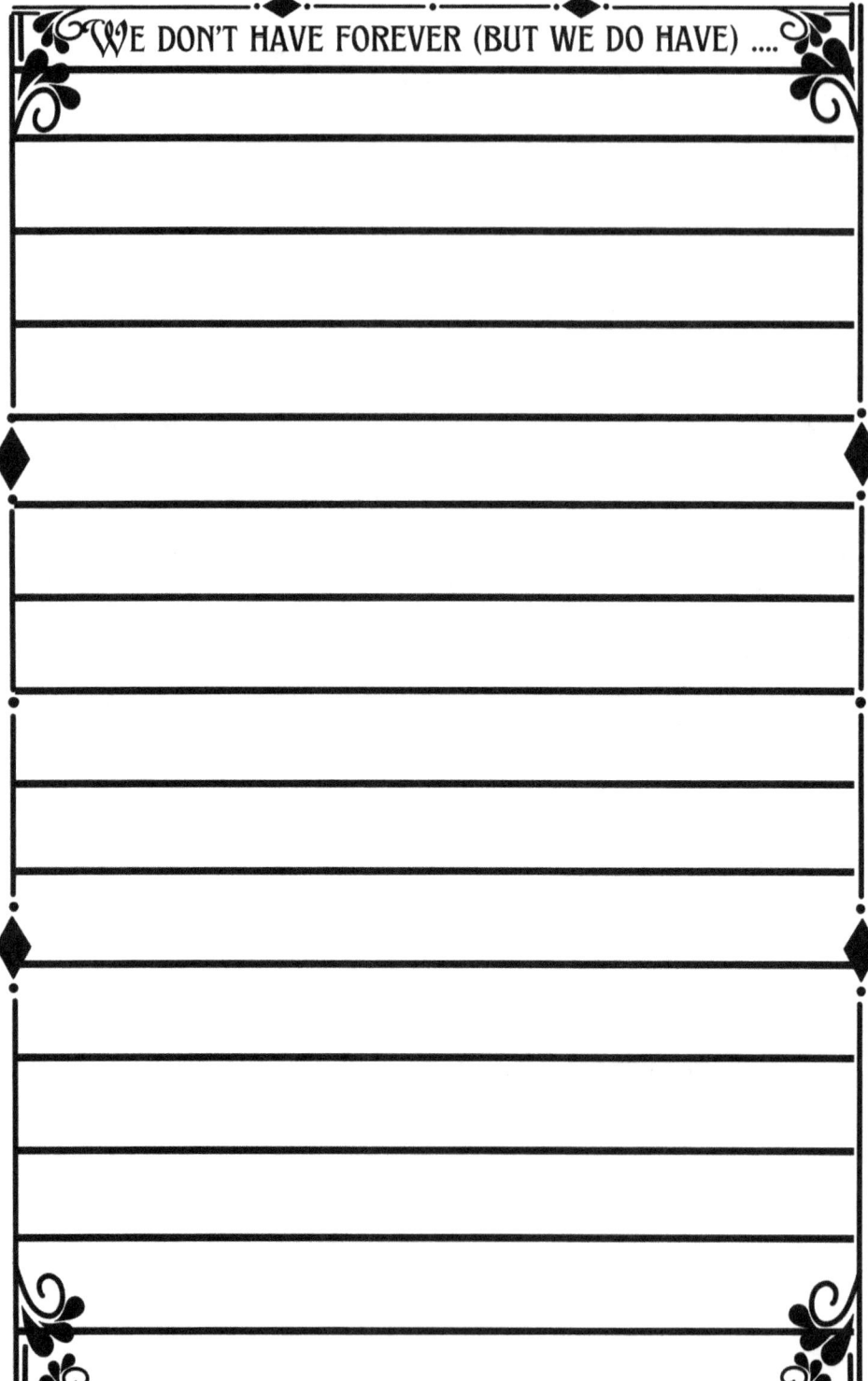

WE DON'T HAVE FOREVER (BUT WE DO HAVE) ....

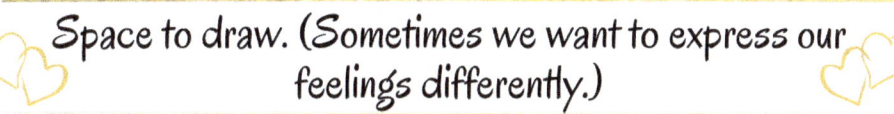

Space to draw. (Sometimes we want to express our feelings differently.)

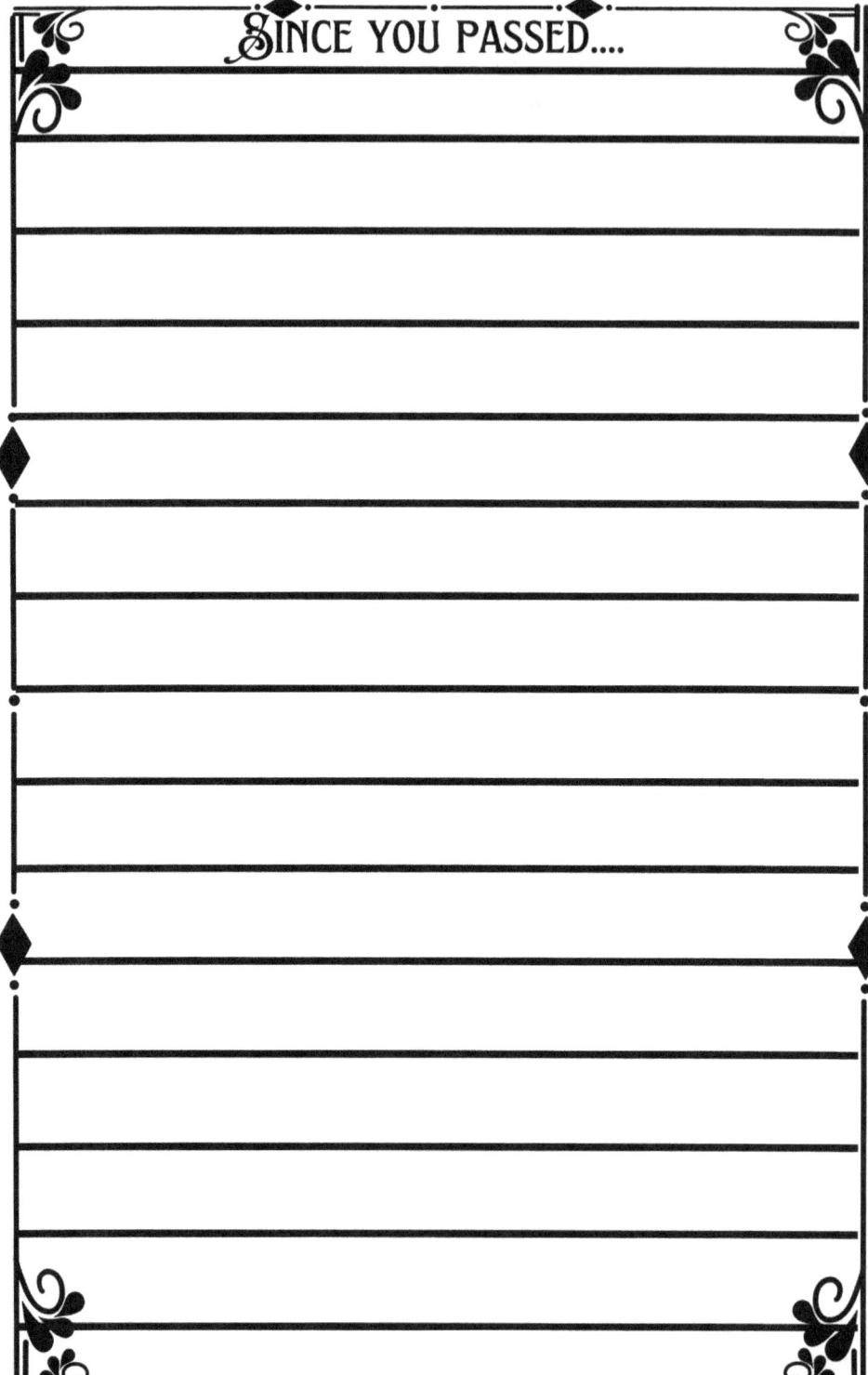

SINCE YOU PASSED....

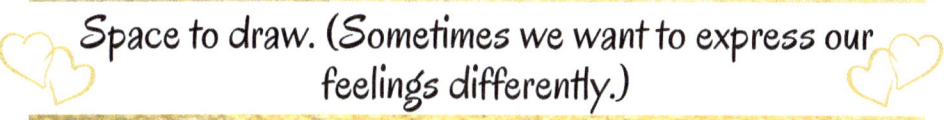

Space to draw. (Sometimes we want to express our feelings differently.)

CREATING PEACE

I had made peace with it long before this moment.

That I had no idea where Athena's grandpa shirt was.

She found a "my little pony" shirt that made her so excited and my heart said "wear it. Grandpa would love to see you this happy" and if he was here, he would tell me to let her wear what she wants and it's no big deal. Nothing over their happiness.

But then as we were ready to go out the door. Athena sees us all, And she says "where's my grandpa shirt?"

Then I went in a panic. Searching the places, I had already searched. Making messes in the spaces I once cleaned.

Found myself ready to cry and even heard myself yell "just look for it. Help me!"

I know this is grief.

Sneaking up on me.

Showing up in ways I wanted to be "better than" but instead got reminded how human I am.

Found a huge shirt.

Put it on Athena.

Used a hair tie to kind of make it work.

And now, we are ready to go. (Only to see Athena moved the flags we had set aside for the cemetery, that I've saved for a month now) the emotions come in quick waves

Juan Ayala your cologne is sprayed.

And My brother just paid for some of todays celebration.

My heart is filled while broken

July 2, 2022

(10/12/22)
Grief is so crazy.

How one moment I can hold hours of conversation of everything hard.
and another moment I can't speak a coupl ofe words without uncontrollable tears and deep breaths.

One moment I can smile with the pain.
and another I can't find any reason to smile.

WHAT ABOUT GRIEF MAKES YOU SMILE? WHAT MAKES YOU CRY?

Tough morning cross guarding. Keeping my feelings in check.

Keeping the tears from releasing.

Saying Good morning to all the beautiful people, when it hurt me to say good morning and yet brought so much gratitude.

Thinking of the shooting in Texas yesterday, it's like I can't not think about it. About them. Their faces.

Someone walked them to school yesterday...said see you later or goodbye or good morning.

That moment in time must have been terrifying and painful.

I hope the day was filled with smiles before it wasn't. Who knows what day each person was having, before that horrible situation took place.

We know some celebrated ceremonies and awards just hours before.

Some dressed up and many looked forward to summer just days or even moments away.

I can't stop the thoughts.
As I woke up this morning to get my family ready for my son's 5th grade graduation, it is very conflicting feelings of fear and gratitude, sadness and excitement.
Yes, all these feelings are present for me.

But it's been a tough morning. To process and move with life, as others' lives have stopped, turned upside down and changed.

For some it's a good morning.
I am thankful to be here.
I am grieving for those lost and hurting.

If you need today to be "normal", it's ok.

If you are numb to this by now
If it's too overwhelming
If it's a good day for you, today....
—— it's ok
Feel your feelings
Be with your journey
Live your life
It's ok to be human
Holding it all

The anger, grief, confusion, rage, gratitude, anxiety, pain, fear, — all of it

— today is tough
And as a collective we have to create change
May 25, 2022

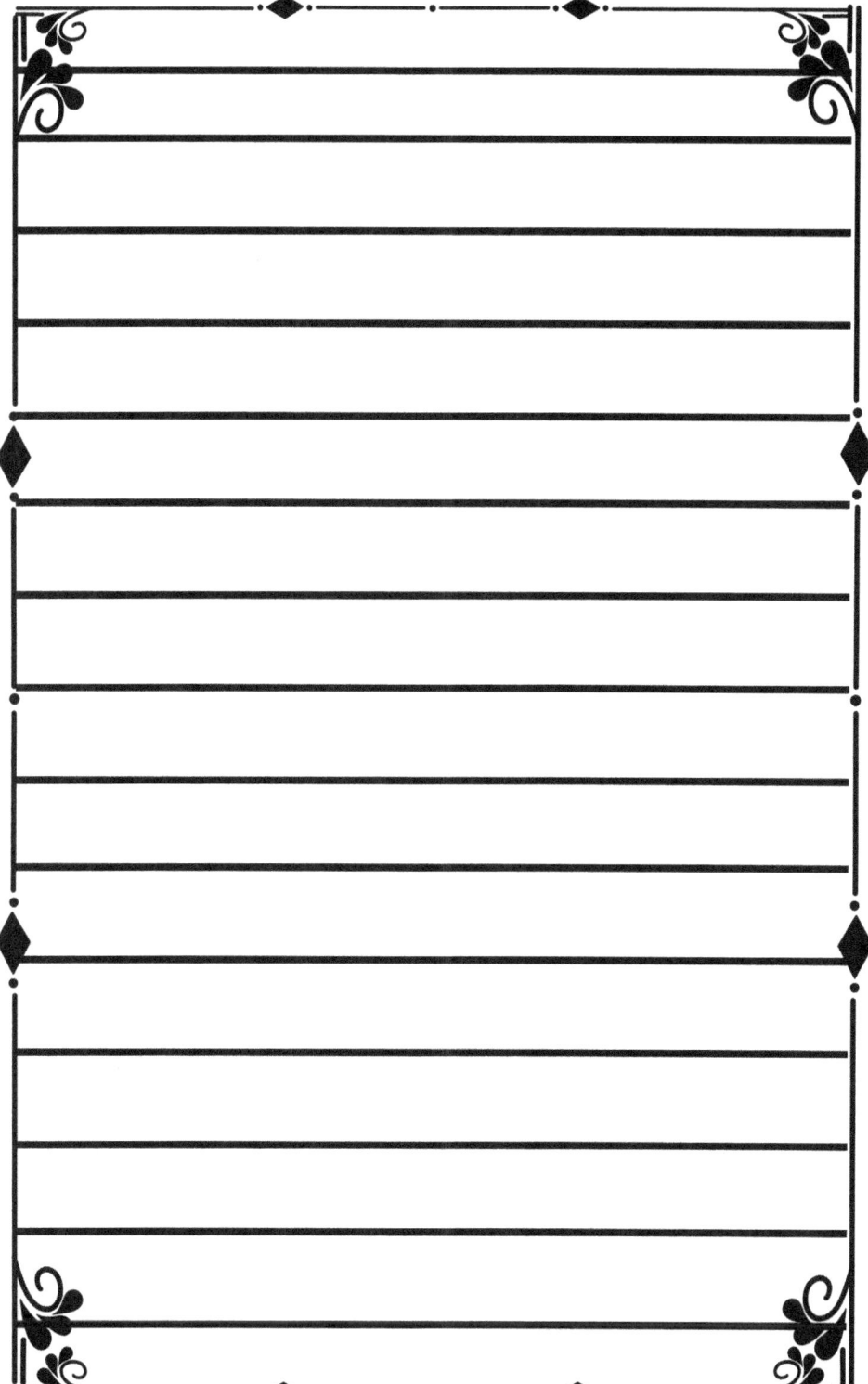

Lena Ayala-Velasquez

Shared with Your friends
11/1/22

Hello soul sister. Can you please send me one of your poetry books
Healing while hurting.
Then I will have all the books you have written. I'm thinking of u during this difficult time. You are "

What a beautiful message to wake up to. To wake up to a reminder of people who I've been blessed to cross paths with and build community with.
a reminder that I am living a dream come true as an author.
a reminder that income is available in different forms.

A reminder that I am making a difference in this world

a reminder that the memory of my dad continues to live on and reach more people

a reminder that the universe has my back

a reminder of gratitude

a reminder to smile, get outside and give thanks

WHAT REMINDER ARE YOU THANKFUL FOR TODAY?

A PIECE OF PEACE (IN THE REALITY)

SOMETIMES BEING THERE FOR OTHERS IN THEIR GRIEF MEANS NOT TREATING THEM DIFFERENTLY. AND JUST BEING YOU WITH THEM.

BABYSITTING WHEN THEY ASK AND LETTING THEM BE WHO AND HOW THEY NEED TO BE IN THIS MOMENT. ALLOWING THAT TO ALL TO BE HERE, PRESENT AND OK

SEPTEMBER 4, 2022

10/21/22

Remembering when I first lost my dad- I am seeing my loved ones do things I used to/and still do

like spray cologne, you gave- just to be reminded of you.

touch your hair and skin-

afraid soon the feeling will feel different.

we started doing things before you were even in hospice care

like we made pillows and altars and said prayers.

we made bears with your voice; you helped make that happen

I took intentional videos and pictures, wanting to hold on to moments.

wanting to hold on to memories

wanting to remember everything.

I almost feel like we were in some ways prepared with my dad

not fully or the same but man.

You can write a whole book and grief and still
not handle situations any "better"
you can write a whole journal for grief, and still
go through it like you have never.
no matter how much you want to be prepared,
you can never be
no matter how much you've been through, you
will go through it all again, differently.
because no situation is ever the same
and pain will always be pain.

learned from loss before, how to be more
present
still trying to better prepare for future by doing
things "different"
and yet grief comes rushing in the same
there's no preparation that can take it away.
just have to feel the feelings
just have to allow what's real to be a part of the
healing.
even when it hurts
because it will always hurt.

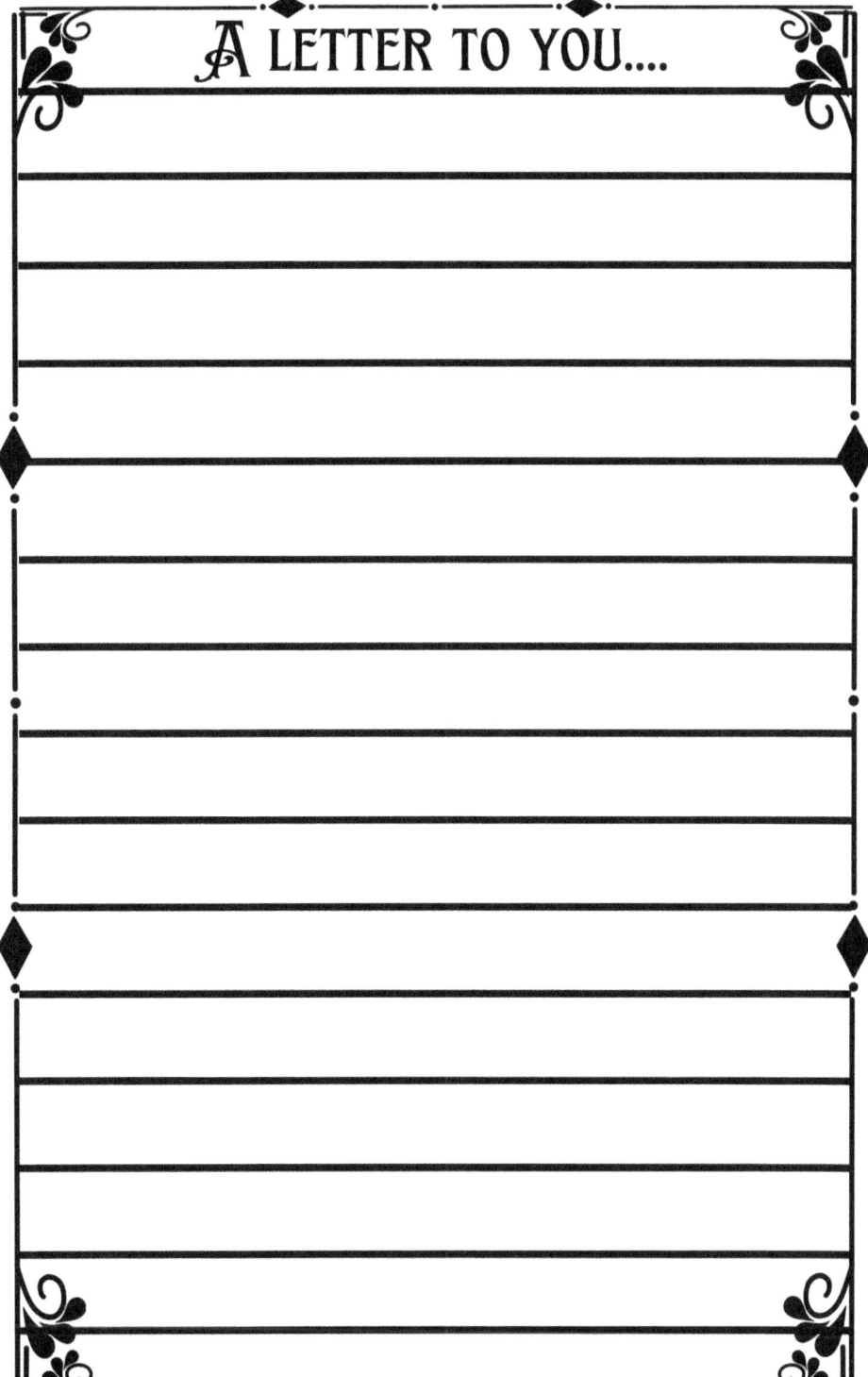

A LETTER TO YOU....

Draw Something

IF YOU KNEW YOU WERE GOING TO LOSE SOMEONE TOMORROW. WHAT WOULD YOU WANT TO REMEMBER?

They say it's grandparents' day. I acknowledge it but that's it. Feels sad. Feels incomplete. While held in gratitude

Our children will only know one of their grandfathers from us as parents, and he has been in heaven for more than a handful of years now.
our children have our two mothers still, one is fighting a tough fight with cancer.

I myself don't even know stories of my parents' fathers. and I only know stories of their mothers, a few picture memories with my mom's mom. Middle names of my grandmothers.
I have grandparents I grew up with. my grandpa Robert and grandma Katie.

My grandma whom I still have in this lifetime. They are my dad's uncle/aunt and godparents but will forever be my grandparents.

my husband has his grandfather on his mom's side still alive but no relationship. pictures of his grandmother on his mom's side but no memories. and no knowledge of grandparents from his father's side, he doesn't even know his father.

so, this day is filled with so much reflection, grief, gratitude and more.

September 11, 2022

NEVER REALLY GONE......BUT ALSO NOT HERE...

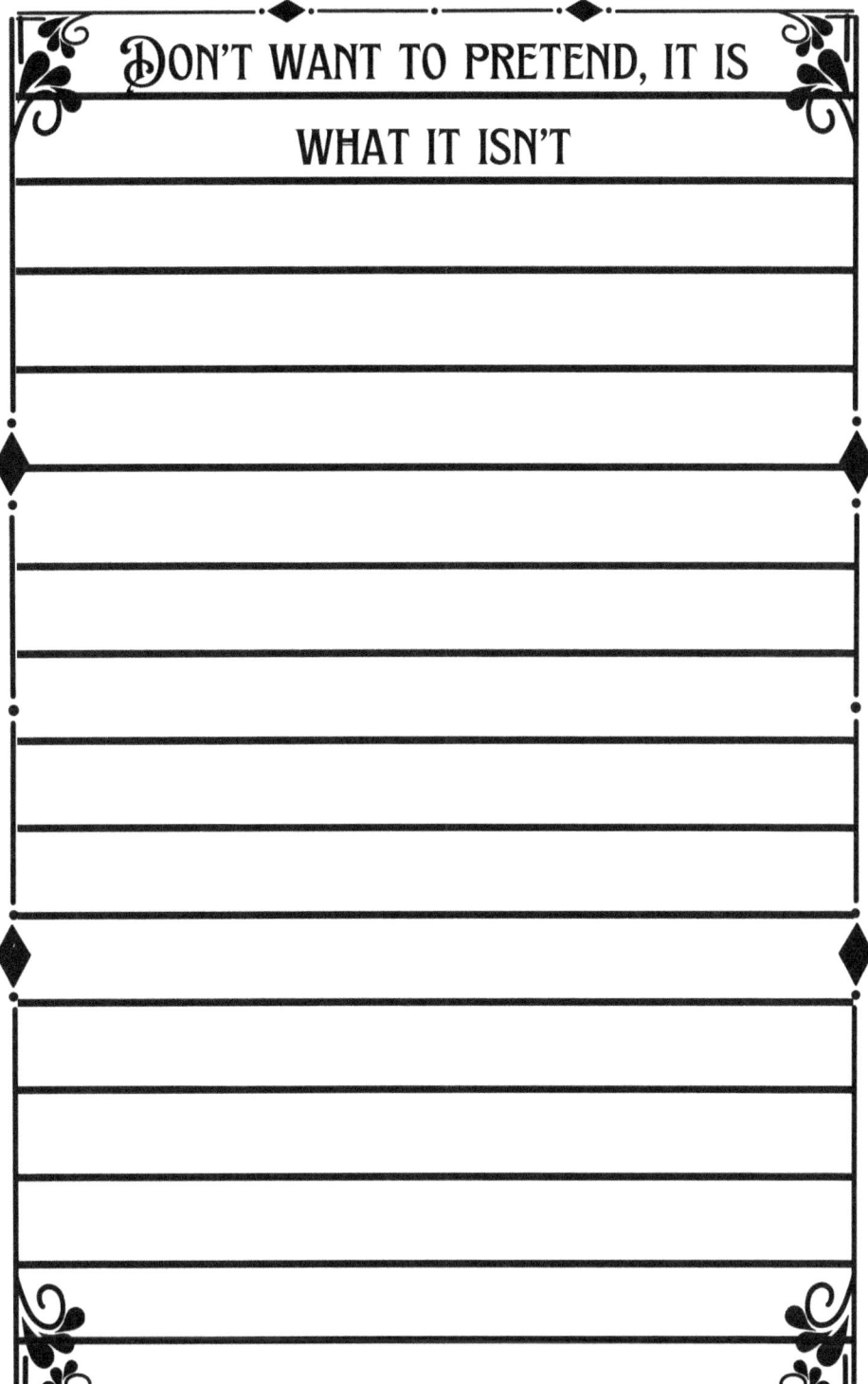

Don't want to pretend, it is what it isn't

Draw Something

THIS IS MY JOURNEY, AND I AM ALLOWING IT....

Draw Something

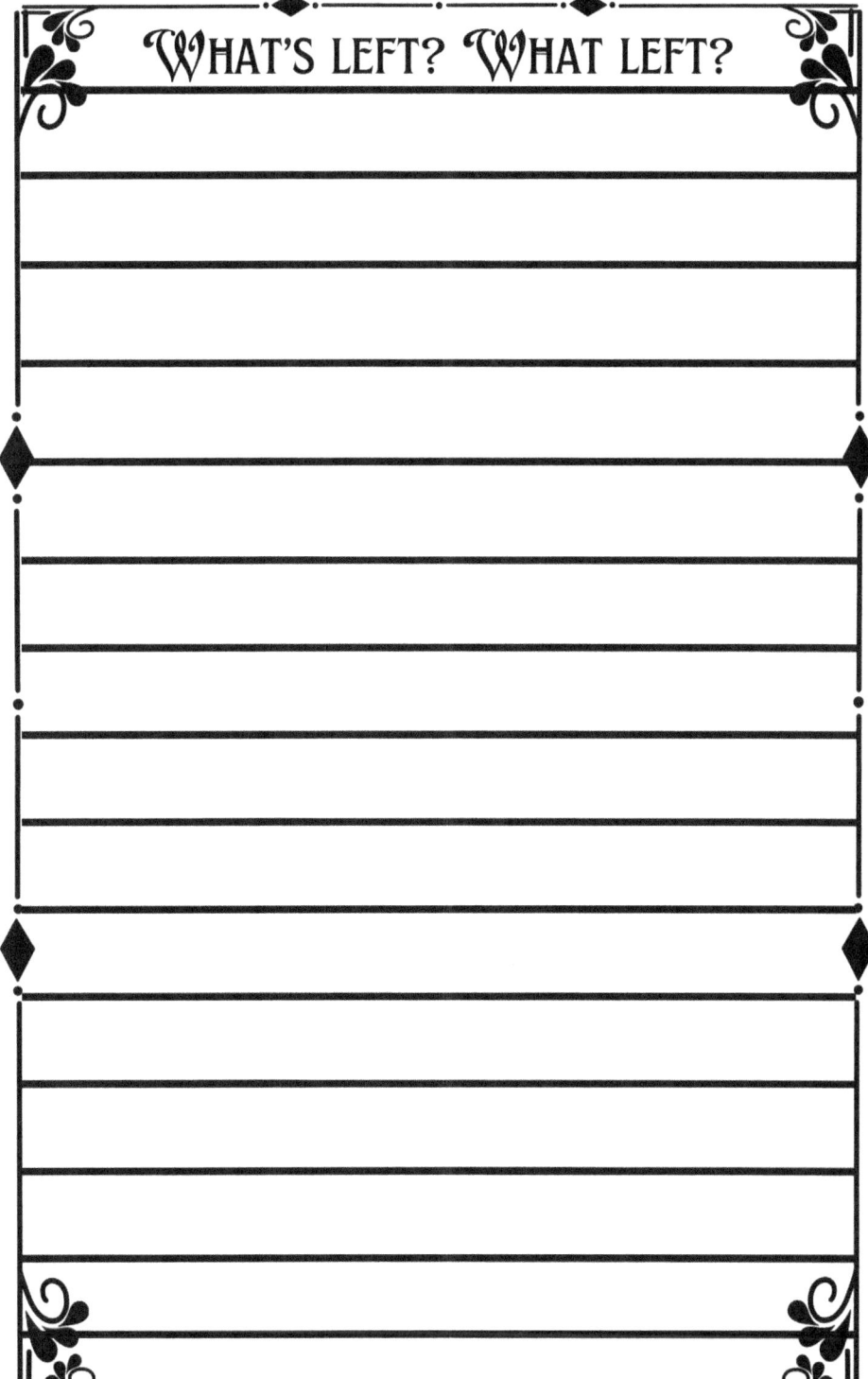

WHAT'S LEFT? WHAT LEFT?

Draw Something

Acknowledgment

When there's too much to lose, no need to prove point of view.

right now, I feel the anger in me rising.
I want to say what I have to say.
I want to stand for what is right.
I want to put people in their place.
I want to defend and protect those I love.
I want to not bite my tongue. I don't want to hold on to this anger or unspoken or hurt.

but it is not the time. I respect that.
I understand enough to know right now is a time that is hard for all. and maybe these situations and reactions are out of emotions that are in grief.
so, I let it be.
no doubt though of the reality that is real within me.
however, I can find peace.

It's unfortunate for anything to happen right now at a time like this.

a time when togetherness should be what's important.

I try to look from outside, why is this happening?

is it a test of us individually and us as a whole?

is it a warning?

is it just what is?

and we go back to, release and move on.

now is not the time.

and yet it is.

but it isn't.

and we make peace with that.

moving on.......

October 22, 2022

IT'S OK TO HEAL. THAT DOESN'T MEAN THAT LOVE IS GONE

FLASHBACKS

Draw Something

WHAT IF

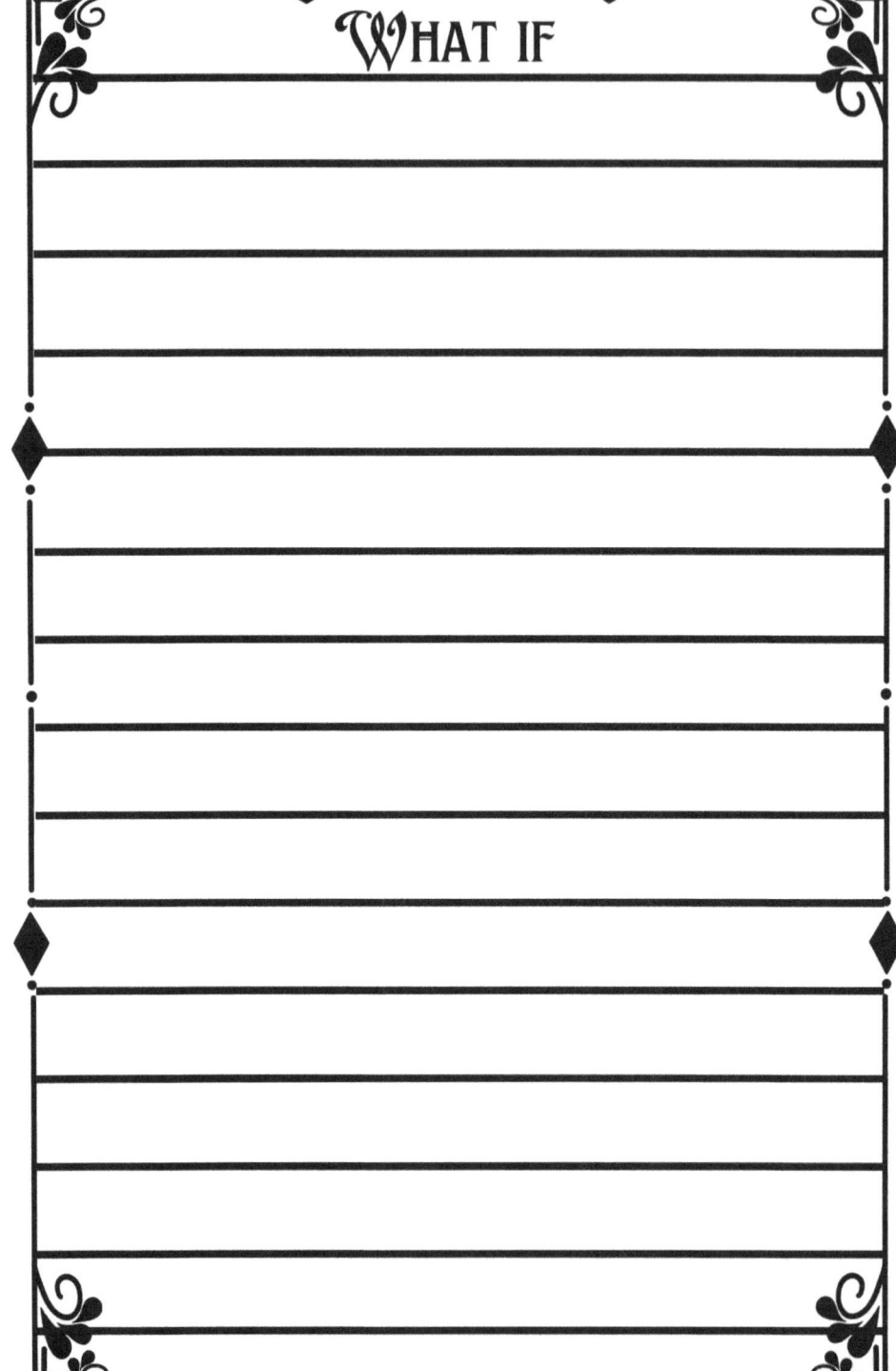

Draw Something

REFLECT ON A HARD SITUATION IN LIFE THAT HELPED SHAPE WHO YOU ARE TODAY. WHAT IS YOUR BIGGEST TAKE-AWAY FROM THAT HARD SITUATION? (QUESTION ASKED.)

January 21, 2014 my dad left this earth physically. There isn't a day, month , year or moment that has gone by where that transition didn't somehow affect me and my life, in too many ways to name.

It is a situation that continues to be a challenge and continues to teach me, guide me and journey with me.

In 2020, my soul told me it was time. Time to write a book about my journey of grief and gratitude. And it was this year where I became a first time self-published author.

Too many lessons learned, some that still come to me even now.

I always knew I would one day be an official author, I never knew until 2020 that this particular journey would be what would be created and make me an author officially.

Some lessons learned:

*That you can write a book that doesn't neccesiarly have an ending.

*Gratitude continues to save me. Even when in one of the hardest parts of my life.

*That it is ok to not be ok. And, it is ok to be ok.

*That my story matters.

*To follow your soul, because it knows what you can't even yet begin to imagine sometimes

*That peace doesn't need to come from picking up the pieces or putting pieces back together. Peace can simply come from being real, authentic, unpolished and true to your heart.

*That people want to hear you

*and that, it is always just the beginning
thank you chelsie for day 4 of your Nourish & Flourish 5-day challenge

September 22, 2022

IT IS OK, TO NOT BE OK.... (WHAT'S NOT OK?)

ARE YOU OKAY? WHAT'S GOING "OK"?

Draw Something

THIS IS HOW I HEAL....

I JUST WANT ANOTHER "LAST"...

Hey dad

hey dad, I know you've been here with us- and with Martha. I know you both have the people you needed and need in heaven to help guide your way.

I know it wasn't easy leaving this world but making your peace with it. Two grandparents and parents now united in this way. On this journey.

You are so very missed down here. But we see the signs that souls live beyond the bodies.

I know you heard me and Edgardo at the cemetery Saturday.

To help guide and support Martha as she now joined you yesterday. (Monday)

Love you both so much. My dad
And my mother-in-law/sponsor/mom.

Only GOD knows the plans but I am so thankful for the awareness and insights we do get to know and believe.

Thank you both for Everything you were and will forever be.
This grief journey is no easy road.
But I will hold you both in realness, gratitude, celebration and faith.

Forever "healing while hurting "
October 25, 2022

SHADOWED BY PAIN....

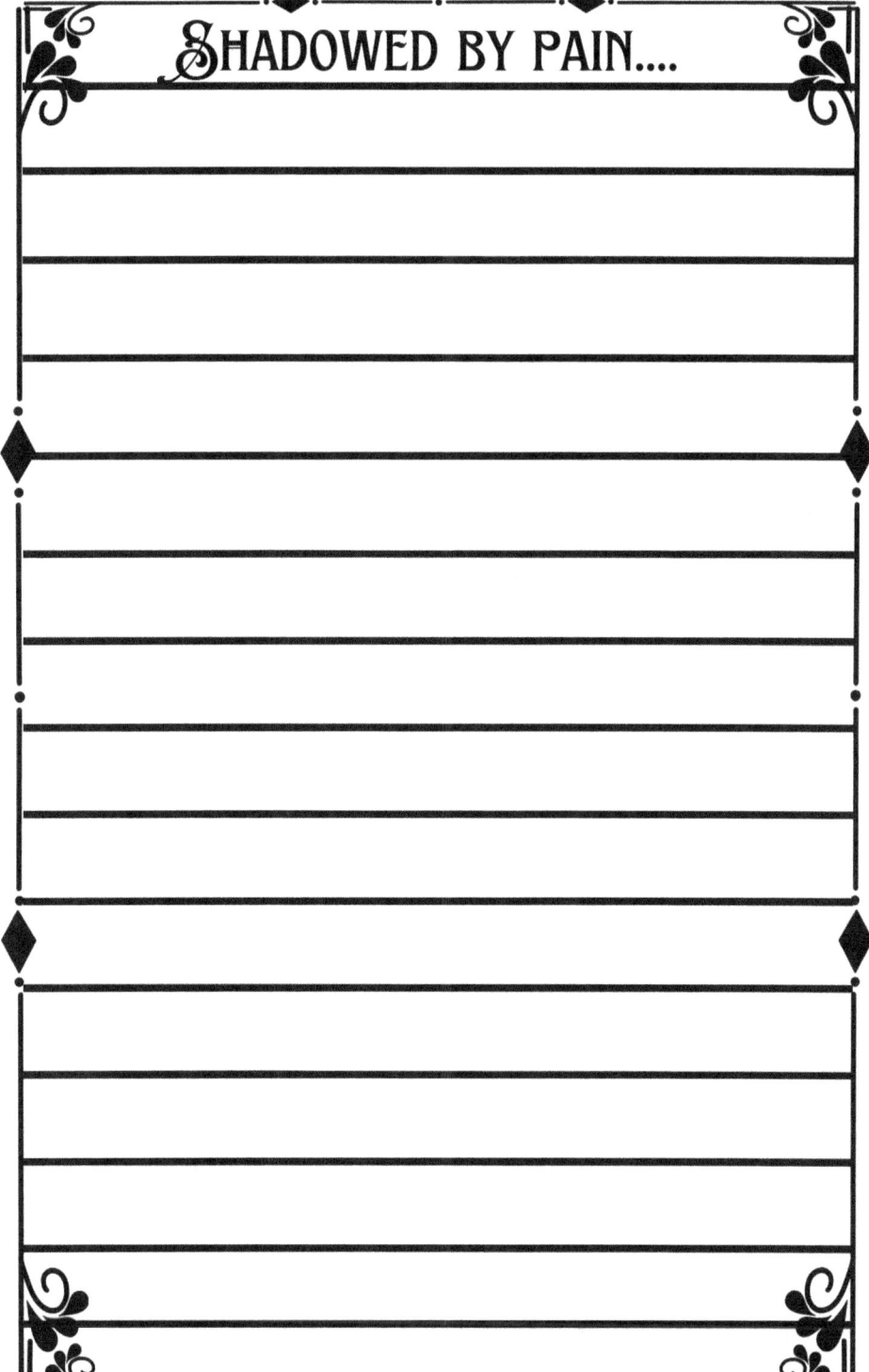

1/12/23

What do I want?

I want to finish writing my book.
I want to complete the upload process.
I want it available for my dad's anniversary.
I want to honor him.
I want to feel like I followed my heart.
I want to serve others.
I want to create income.
I want to feel good.
I want to make my family proud.
I want to see my dream come true.
I want to live in my purpose
I want to live a life I love.

When it's personal, it's following my heart. It will lead to what I can build from. It fulfills me.

WHAT DO YOU WANT?

THIS HOSPICE CARE IS A NEW
JOURNEY FOR ME.
FLASHBACKS OF MY DAD'S
TRANSITION- ALTHOUGH IT
HAPPENED DIFFERENTLY.
GRIEF AND GRATITUDE.

OCTOBER 18, 2022

I believe like the rain and sun have to come together to form a rainbow, that we are human and that life is so much better when you are able to embrace the beauty and the struggles. For me, it is true that those things often go hand in hand (the rain and the sun) you don't really have one without the other. Life is all about how you look at it. What you make of it. We are indeed in charge of our choices.

We can be in charge of creating new thoughts which lead to creating new actions. We can live happier and healthier life. Stress is damaging but we can choose differently. I believe so much in gratitude. I am learning as an adult, the benefits of gratitude and living abundantly. I have always known these things to be true but now I have different education, experiences, and knowledge to further support me so I can help others.

WHAT ARE YOU GRATEFUL FOR?

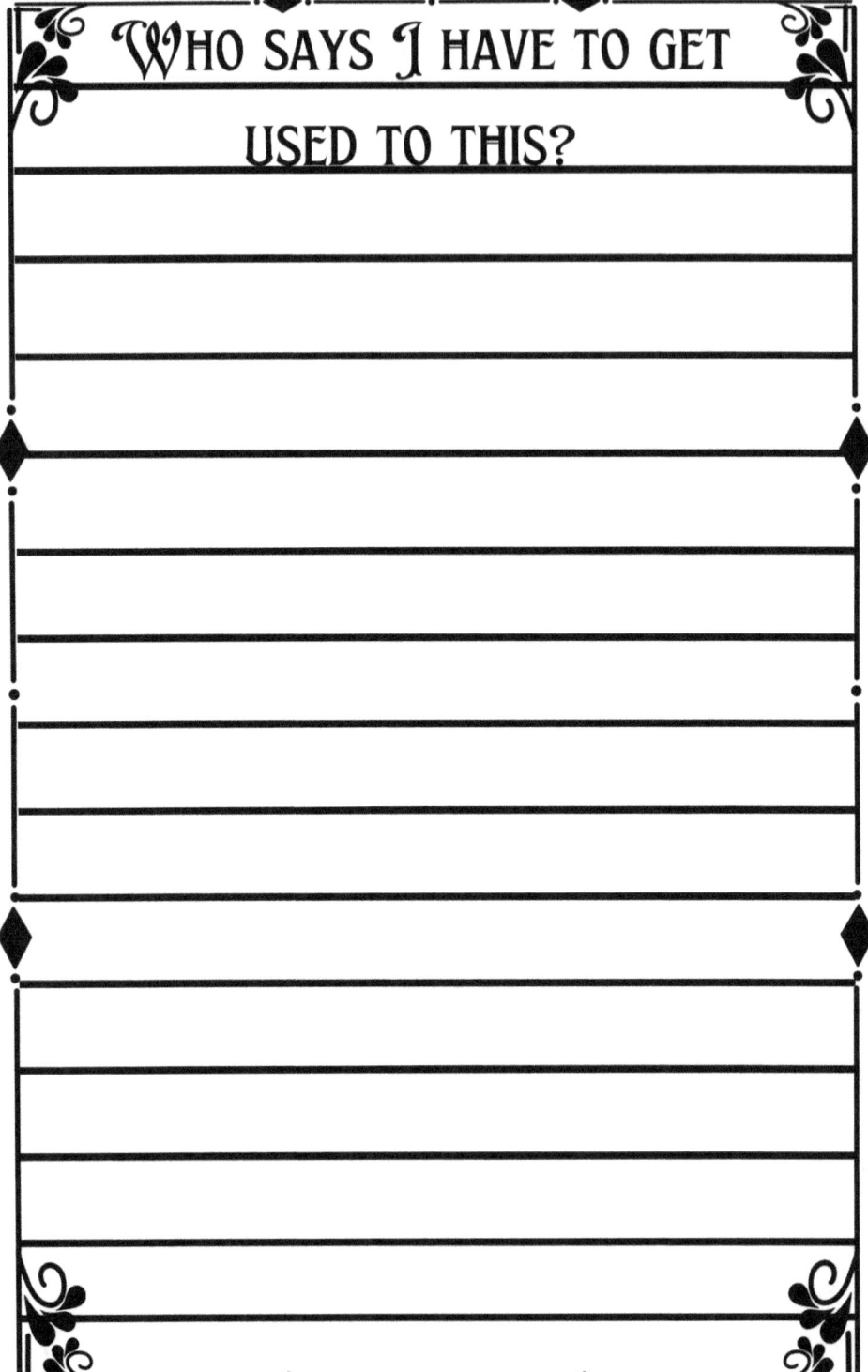

WHO SAYS I HAVE TO GET USED TO THIS?

HOW DO YOU GRIEVE?

IT DOESN'T HAVE TO MEAN GRIEVING WITH DEATH.

IT CAN MEAN GRIEF OF ANY KIND (LIKE MOVING, A BREAKUP, SOMETHING YOU LOVE BREAKING OR BEING LOST OR STOLEN.
IT CAN BE A DREAM THAT HASN'T COME TRUE OR ONE THAT ENDED. IT CAN BE ANYTHING THAT IS TRUE FOR YOU. (SOME EXAMPLES OF HOW I DEAL WITH GRIEF ARE: I PRAY, GO TO THE CEMETERY, TALK TO OTHERS, JOURNAL, EAT FOODS THAT MAKE ME HAPPY, LOOK AT PICTURES, LISTEN TO MUSIC, CRY....)

THERE IS NO WRONG ANSWER.

WHAT CAN YOU LET GO OF TO MAKE SPACE FOR MORE OF WHAT YOU WANT?

TRANSITIONS

I always say what December/Christmas time is to many- October is to me/us.
Well, October this year was a lot of heartache.
A lot of extra financial hardship.
So much struggle and challenge and trauma on so many levels. Spiritually, mentally, emotionally, physically.

October is a month of many birthdays: including mine, our daughter who turned the special 15 and our son who turned 16.

My mother-in-law transitioned October 24....
not only that but spent over a month in the hospital prior and then about 10 days in hospice.
so, it was a long journey. A new journey for us all.
and here we are November 20th and we are still finding our way through processing and accepting and life.

we made peace with October and birthdays not being what we once wanted birthdays to be.
we were and still are in our grief. and that is ok.

well today, debt doesn't end. Life is still hard. struggle is still real.
some wishes will never come true and some will still take time and some will become real today.
In this moment of going further into debt, feels scary and so happy. Angel got his ps5! which is hard to find. And thankful to know people who found us one and will let us pay over time.
In this moment I feel like "we are taking back October"

In this moment I feel like why not go into debt for some smiles. we are already in debt for shelter/food/death and lack of self-care.
we have given up so much.

grounded in gratitude through it all, yes. impulsive right now, because we missed several chances of taking the risk and lost out on cheaper deals and opportunity.
not missing out again.
another thing added to the stress list. but this one comes with some smiles and some happy tears.
this one comes with some motivation for us all.
take back your happiness. whether that be materialistic, or not.

Take it back. and be with what brings you some joy.

because having joy is so important. to your whole well-being.

what's next? we are coming for you.

thank you, community. thank you credit cards.

hoping black Friday deals come in supportive. hoping book sales come through.

hoping hard work and faith and everything else- works in our favor.

because the hard will always be hard. and there will always be new "hard" when you overcome another.

it's time to go for happy. choose happy.

today, in this moment-"a little late but worth the wait. happy 16th birthday "

——November 20, 2022

1/5/22 ANCESTORS

We ourselves will be someone's ancestors, one day.
what are we teaching those around us, right now?
what are we modeling?
where are we not allowing acceptance and growth and change?
why does our way have to be the only way or the right way?
what anger and pain are we holding?
how is anger and pain leading us?

how is anger and pain holding us back?
what can we learn from our kids?
how can we keep our ancestor's teachings and create new paths for different knowledge and healing?
how can we acknowledge another's story and path, even if we don't agree or choose differently?
how do we live on, even after we are gone?
what ways do you want to live on?
show up in the ways that will allow the version and lessons you truly want to leave behind, to live on.

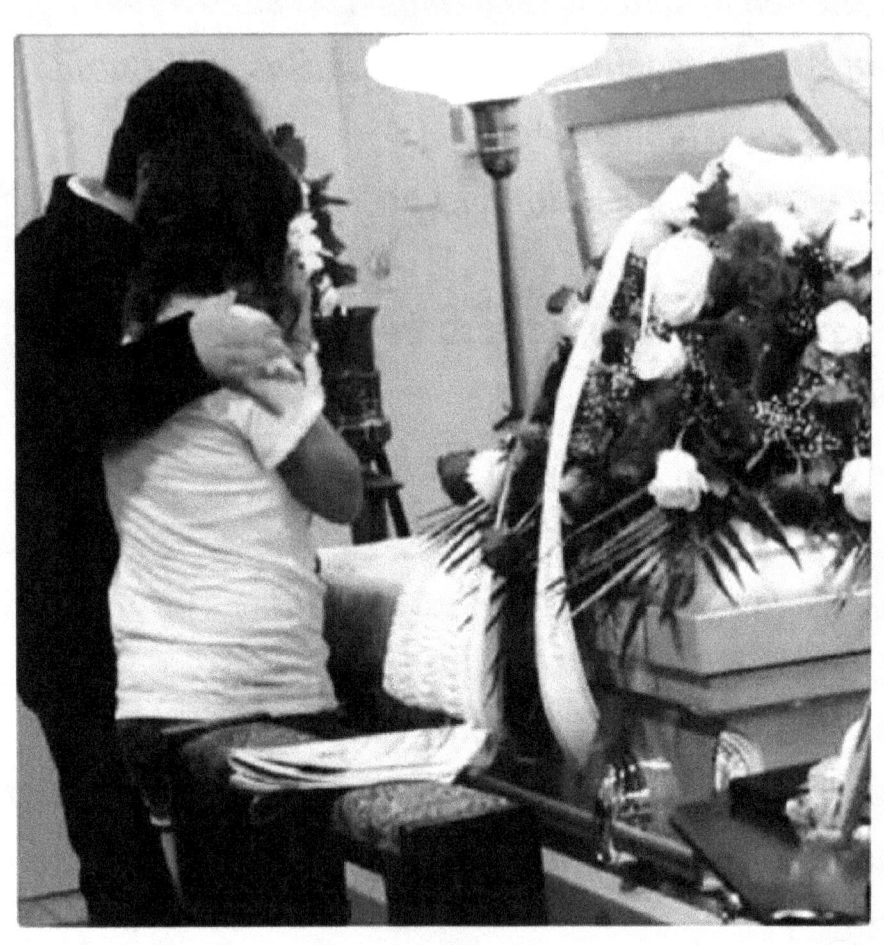

FREE YOURSELF

That fear feels like it's strangling me
stopping me from stepping into my dream.
left me with what if
but too scared to take the risk.

what is the risk?
my heart knows what my purpose and
intention is.
I love to give, so I need to move forward
Others deserve me to step in further.

My words shared are more than just diary
pages written
I am being generous with myself and generous
with others when I write what I have written.
and it goes beyond the pages, because I share it
beyond myself
this is how I live freely, this is how I free
myself.
——1/31/23

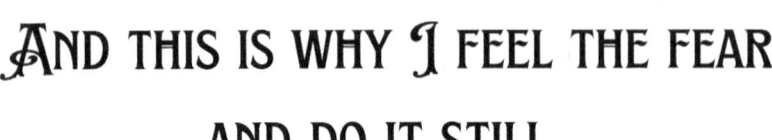

And this is why I feel the fear
and do it still.
For the release. For the peace.
To answer the calls in my heart.

If you don't know when or how,
just start.

Learn your why, and go from
there.
Come back to "why"- every time
and it will take you beyond the
fear.

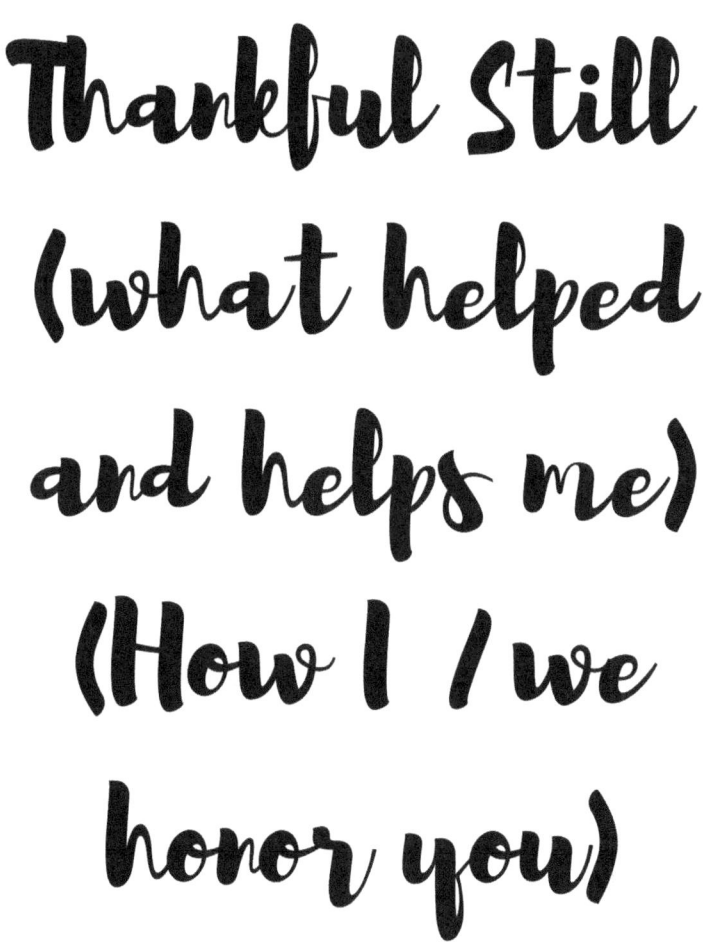

Thankful Still
(what helped
and helps me)
(How I / we
honor you)

Writing has helped me in processing my thoughts and feelings. Writing still supports me when it comes to finding clarity and release. Writing is healing for me.

*Poetry has been an outlet for me since elementary school. Reading it, listening to it and writing it myself.

*Journaling supports me. Taking time to sit with my thoughts, express them through writing online or on paper or on my phone. Sometimes I even record voice messages to myself when I want to write.

*I honor loved ones by talking about them. Sharing memories. Writing about them. Keeping their names spoken. Sharing pictures. Keeping them in our thoughts and celebrations.

*Sometimes honoring looks like going to the cemetery, sometimes it sounds like silent prayers, sometimes it looks like watching old videos. There's no one way. There's no wrong or right way.

*Something that helps me when it comes to grief, is being transparent about it. Being able to speak my truth, even when it doesn't make sense.

*Writing books has helped me in ways that I never even imagined.

*The list goes on and on. But gratitude saved me, time and time again. I don't know where I would be if I didn't allow myself to feel my feelings and turn to gratitude in partnership

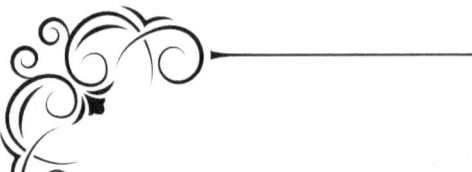

Grateful Though (What I Have Learned~What I Wish I Knew)

*I have learned that grief has no end. It is an on-going journey

*I have learned that life insurance is important.
When your family is left without financial help, it can be very hard and stressful to come up with the finances to provide a funeral of any kind, especially one that you may feel your loved one deserves.

*Creating a gofundme can be extrmeley helpful. It can generate a large amount of money and quickly.

*Prices for everything, including death and funerals have gone up.

*I have learned you have the option to watch your loved one be burried. To watch the actual dirt be placed upon the casket.

*I wish I knew exactly what loved ones wanted for themselves once they were gone

I wish I asked : What do you want us to know or do?
Do you want to be burried or creamated, or something else?
Do you have an outfit in mind?
Do you have a final resting spot chosen, or that you would love most?

Blessed Always
(Thank You,
About Me)

I like to end my days with reflecting on my daily gratitudes. I feel it's only right to end this journal, with some thank you's.

Thank you, for supporting my author journey by having this journal in your hands. Thank you for taking time to read or write, or participate in both. Thank you for taking time to reflect, to dig deeper, to process, to share this space with me. I hope you remember that you can restart any time and as many times as you feel the desire to.

As I said in my book (Pandemic poetry and reflections) Gratitude always helps me. It helps me know life is always great and helps me see through the struggle differently.

Gratitude through my body, feels neccesary for me. It feels like: more calm, more peace, literally.

We can't redo what can't be redone. We can't replace what's lost or gone. In grief and gratitude- it's accepted. Trying to embrace while allowing the broken pieces.
-Oct 31, 22

Grief and celebration can coexist. They do. With or without permission. But that permission part can make a difference.
-September 24, 22

A LITTLE BIT ABOUT ME, THE CREATOR OF THIS BOOK/JOURNAL.

THIS BOOK IS MY 6TH SELF-PUBLISHED BOOK.

- HEALING WHILE HURTING, POETRY AND REFLECTIONS.
- RATCHET GRANDMA: WHO'S BABYSITTING WHO? (NOT FOR SALE TO THE PUBLIC).
- PANDEMIC POETRY AND REFLECTIONS.
- GRATITUDE SAVED ME, JOURNAL PROMPTS, AND REFLECTIONS.
- DIARY OF A CROSSING GUARD, STARGELL AND MOSLEY.
- HEALING WHILE WRITING, JOURNAL PROMPTS, AND REFLECTIONS.

My name is Carolina but to many I am Lena. I am a wife, a mother and former yet forever teacher. I realized in my thirties I had pieces of me outside of being a wife, mom and teacher that still wanted to be lived.

So, I allowed myself to dream again and go after those dreams - step by step until they became the life I was living. Being an author is one of those dream come true's and it's a constant source of gratitude and happiness. I truly believe I am living my life's purpose each time I allow myself to follow my heart. .

No-matter the title certain positions or situations hold. Right now I am enjoying being a crossing guard and self-published author. I enjoy being in charge of my stories, telling my truths and the journey each book is taking me on.

Each book has it's own story of how it became real. Each book has had it's own process. Each book teaches me so much about myself and this journey. Each book is different levels of healing for me and so many layers of my life, my heart.

ALLOW YOURSELF TO
DREAM.
THEN, JUST TAKE THE
NEXT STEP.
OVER AND OVER
AGAIN.

I am not a therapist or doctor or trying to convince you what to do or how to live. I am just a person sharing my stories, journey, truth, and experiences. I am not telling you what to do or believe. I am not saying what you should or shouldn't do. I do not believe what works for one person, works for all. We are all different.

What's true for me is that grief and gratitude can co-exist and often do. It is up to us whether we permit them to be real together or if we treat them as separate pieces. If you leave with anything I hope you were able to dig deeper, reflect, be true to yourself, and invite in time to reflect, get creative, and just be.

Maxine Sanchez, and Larry Aragon

A service will be held at the Chapel of Roses, 1940 Peralta Blvd, Fremont, at 11:00am on Jan 25, 2014.

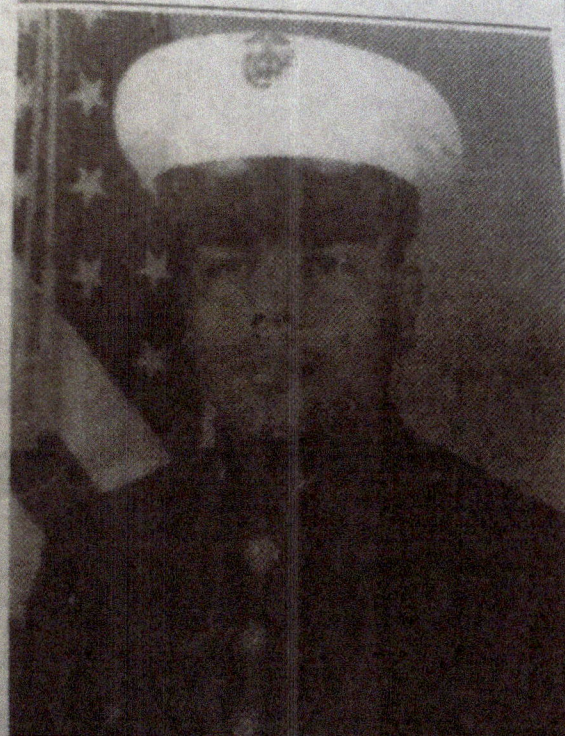

Juan R. Ayala
July 2, 1961 - January 21, 2014
Resident of Fremont

Entered into rest on

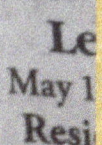

Le
May 1
Resi

Leon
in Jan
(Nuszl
Cisek
Polan
in th
twelft
in a
ily, h
schoo
Churc
then
Schoo
1955,
Metca

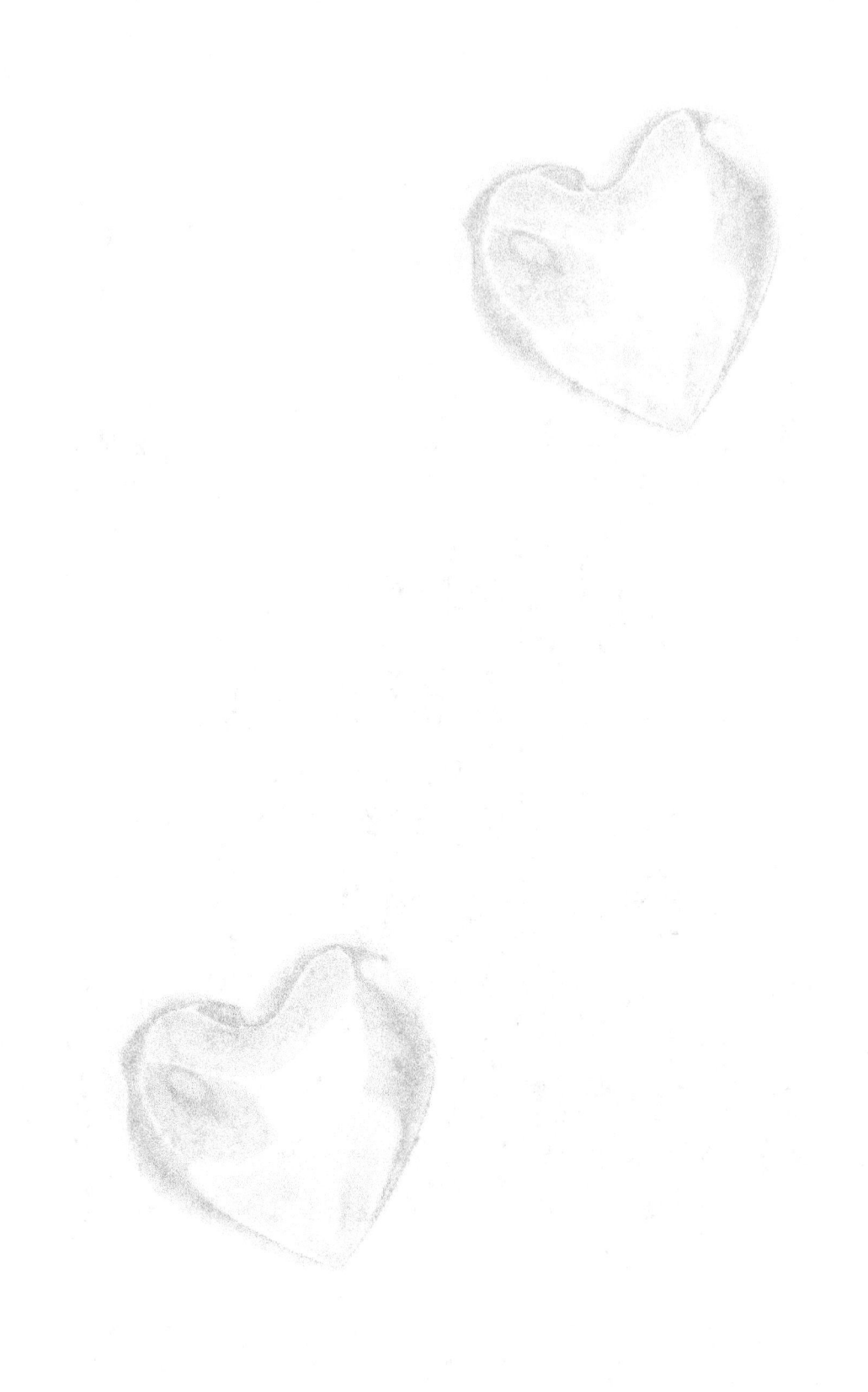

www.ingramcontent.com/pod-product-compliance
Lightning Source LLC
Chambersburg PA
CBHW071146130626
46553CB00004B/1541